T0259518

Feedlot Processing and Arrival Cattle Management

Editors

BRAD J. WHITE
DANIEL U. THOMSON

VETERINARY CLINICS OF NORTH AMERICA: FOOD ANIMAL PRACTICE

www.vetfood.theclinics.com

Consulting Editor
ROBERT A. SMITH

July 2015 • Volume 31 • Number 2

ELSEVIER

1600 John F. Kennedy Boulevard • Suite 1800 • Philadelphia, Pennsylvania, 19103-2899

http://www.vetfood.theclinics.com

VETERINARY CLINICS OF NORTH AMERICA: FOOD ANIMAL PRACTICE Volume 31, Number 2
July 2015 ISSN 0749-0720, ISBN-13: 978-0-323-39123-8

Editor: Patrick Manley
Developmental Editor: Meredith Clinton

Veterinary Clinics of North America: Food Animal Practice (ISSN 0749-0720) is published in March, July, and November by Elsevier Inc., 360 Park Avenue South, New York, NY 10010-1710. Subscription prices are $235.00 per year (domestic individuals), $326.00 per year (domestic institutions), $110.00 per year (domestic students/residents), $265.00 per year (Canadian individuals), $430.00 per year (Canadian institutions), $335.00 per year (international individuals), $430.00 per year (international institutions), and $165.00 per year (international and Canadian students/residents). To receive student/resident rate, orders must be accompanied by name of affiliated institution, date of term, and the signature of program/residency coordinator on institution letterhead. *Clinics* subscription prices. All prices are subject to change without notice. **POSTMASTER:** Send address changes to *Veterinary Clinics of North America*: *Food Animal Practice*, Elsevier Health Sciences Division, Subscription Customer Service, 3251 Riverport Lane, Maryland Heights, MO 63043. Customer Service (orders, claims, online, change of address): Elsevier Health Sciences Division, Subscription **Customer Service, 3251 Riverport Lane, Maryland Heights, MO 63043. Tel: 1-800-654-2452 (U.S. and Canada); 314-447-8871 (ouside U.S. and Canada). Fax: 314-447-8029. E-mail: journalscustomerservice-usa@elsevier.com (for print support); journalsonlinesupport-usa@elsevier.com (for online support).**

Reprints. For copies of 100 or more, of articles in this publication, please contact the Commercial Reprints Department, Elsevier Inc., 360 Park Avenue South, New York, NY 10010-1710. Tel.: 212-633-3874; Fax: 212-633-3820; E-mail: reprints@elsevier.com.

Veterinary Clinics of North America: Food Animal Practice is covered in *Current Contents/Agriculture, Biology and Environmental Sciences, MEDLINE/PubMed (Index Medicus), and Excerpta Medica.*

Contributors

CONSULTING EDITOR

ROBERT A. SMITH, DVM, MS
Diplomate, American Board of Veterinary Practitioners; Veterinary Research and Consulting Services, LLC, Greeley, Colorado

EDITORS

BRAD J. WHITE, DVM, MS
Department of Clinical Sciences, College of Veterinary Medicine, Kansas State University, Manhattan, Kansas

DANIEL U. THOMSON, DVM, PhD
Department of Diagnostic Medicine and Pathobiology, College of Veterinary Medicine, Kansas State University, Manhattan, Kansas

AUTHORS

MICHAEL D. APLEY, DVM, PhD
Diplomate, American College of Veterinary Clinical Pharmacology; Frick Professor, Department of Clinical Sciences, College of Veterinary Medicine, Kansas State University, Manhattan, Kansas

PAUL BECK, PhD
Department of Animal Sciences, University of Arkansas, Fayetteville, Arkansas

CALVIN W. BOOKER, DVM, MVetSc
Managing Partner, Feedlot Health Management Services Ltd, Okotoks, Alberta, Canada

TIMOTHY J. GOLDSMITH, DVM, MPH
Diplomate, American College of Veterinary Clinical Pharmacology; Assistant Professor, Center for Animal Health and Food Safety, College of Veterinary Medicine, University of Minnesota, Minneapolis, Minnesota

DEE GRIFFIN, DVM, MS
University of Nebraska-Lincoln, Lincoln, Nebraska; Great Plains Veterinary Educational Center, Clay Center, Nebraska

DANIEL L. GROOMS, DVM, PhD
Professor, Department of Large Animal Clinical Sciences, Michigan State University, East Lansing, Michigan

W. MARK HILTON, DVM
Diplomate, American Board of Veterinary Practitioners (Beef Cattle Practice); Department of Veterinary Clinical Sciences, Purdue University College of Veterinary Medicine, West Lafayette, Indiana

LEE ANNE K. KROLL, DVM, MS
Arenec Bay Veterinary Services, Standish, Michigan

TIFFANY L. LEE, DVM, MS
Graduate Research Assistant, Beef Cattle Institute, Kansas State University, Manhattan, Kansas

TERRY L. MADER, MS, PhD
Professor Emeritus, University of Nebraska-Lincoln, Lincoln, Nebraska

JEREMY POWELL, PhD, DVM
Department of Animal Sciences, University of Arkansas, Fayetteville, Arkansas

RYAN D. RADEMACHER, DVM
Professional Services Veterinarian, Feedlot Health Management Services Ltd, Okotoks, Alberta, Canada

CHRIS REINHARDT, PhD
Extension Feedlot Specialist, Department of Animal Sciences and Industry, College of Agriculture, Kansas State University, Manhattan, Kansas

DAVID N. RETHORST, DVM
Outreach Director, Beef Cattle Institute, College of Veterinary Medicine, Kansas State University, Manhattan, Kansas

ROBERT A. SMITH, DVM, MS
Diplomate, American Board of Veterinary Practitioners; Veterinary Research and Consulting Services, LLC, Greeley, Colorado

GERALD STOKKA, DVM, MS
Associate Professor, Department of Animal Sciences, Extension Veterinarian/Livestock Stewardship, North Dakota State University, Fargo, North Dakota

DANIEL U. THOMSON, DVM, PhD
Department of Diagnostic Medicine and Pathobiology, College of Veterinary Medicine, Kansas State University, Manhattan, Kansas

CHRIS A. TUCKER, PhD
Department of Animal Sciences, University of Arkansas, Fayetteville, Arkansas

BRIAN N. WARR, DVM
Professional Services Veterinarian, Feedlot Health Management Services Ltd, Okotoks, Alberta, Canada

CHRISTINE WEINGARTZ, BS
Department of Animal Sciences, University of Arkansas, Fayetteville, Arkansas

EVA WRAY, BS
Department of Animal Sciences, University of Arkansas, Fayetteville, Arkansas

THOMAS A. YAZWINSKI, PhD
Department of Animal Sciences, University of Arkansas, Fayetteville, Arkansas

Contents

The practice of vaccination has been used for more than 200 years and is an important component of livestock preventive medicine programs. The goal of vaccination is to stimulate an immune response in an individual that will protect that individual from disease or reduce the clinical signs in that individual. Vaccination applied to a population has a similar goal, as well as decreasing or preventing spread within a population. Commercial vaccines are evaluated for efficacy and safety, and the proper application of these products to varied cattle populations requires knowledge of risk factors and production system factors.

When studying the practice of preconditioning (PC) calves, many factors need to be examined to determine if cow-calf producers should make this investment. Factors such as average daily gain, feed efficiency, available labor, length of the PC period, genetics, and marketing options must be analyzed. The health sales price advantage is an additional benefit in producing and selling PC calves, but not the sole determinant of PC's financial feasibility. Studies show that a substantial advantage of PC is the selling of additional pounds at a cost of gain well below the marginal return of producing those additional pounds.

Pregnant heifers in the feedlot pose many economic and management issues to the producer. Heifers that enter the feedlot pregnant will have increased costs associated with them regardless of the management strategy implemented. It is imperative that practitioners be aware of management concerns associated with pregnant heifers in order to provide sound recommendations for their clients. The purpose of this article is to provide the bovine practitioner with a summary of current literature and present common options for managing pregnant heifers in a feedlot setting.

Fly and louse infestations are readily discerned and remedied in feedlot cattle. Tapeworm and fluke infections are accepted as probable but, given

disease include time in transit from their origin, which is likely to be highly correlated with the amount of time away from quality feed and water. A high risk of developing respiratory disease is likely to correlate well with the animals' suppressed appetite immediately after arrival. This article discusses 2 distinctive categories of feeder animals (high-risk calves and yearlings) and their nutritional needs.

Indoor confined feedlots offer advantages that make them desirable in northern climates where high rainfall and snowfall occur. These facilities increase the risk of certain health risks, including lameness and tail injuries. Closed confinement can also facilitate the rapid spread of infectious disease. Veterinarians can help to manage these health risks by implementing management practices to reduce their occurrence.

The days of oral treatment instructions and loosely associated authorizations for the use of drugs in food animals are gone. Treatment protocols should include case definitions for treatment eligibility, detailed regimens, case definitions for treatment success and failure, directions for animal disposition, and mechanisms to prevent animals entering the food chain with violative residues. Prescriptions and veterinary feed directives (VFDs) will soon be necessary for almost all uses of antimicrobials in food animals. Although VFDs have a regulatory format, prescriptions may vary, but there are basic inclusions that should be present in any prescription.

VETERINARY CLINICS OF NORTH AMERICA: FOOD ANIMAL PRACTICE

FORTHCOMING ISSUES

November 2015
Feedlot Production Medicine
Brad J. White and Daniel U. Thomson, *Editors*

March 2016
Update on Ruminant Ultrasound
Sébastien Buczinski, *Editor*

July 2016
Bovine Theriogenology
Robert L. Larson, *Editor*

RECENT ISSUES

March 2015
Bovine Clinical Pharmacology
Michael D. Apley, *Editor*

November 2014
Dairy Nutrition
Robert J. Van Saun, *Editor*

July 2014
Fluid and Electrolyte Therapy
Alan J. Roussel and Geof W. Smith, *Editors*

ISSUE OF RELATED INTEREST

Veterinary Clinics of North America: Small Animal Practice
July 2015 (Vol. 45, Issue 4)
Urology
Joseph W. Bartges, *Editor*

Preface

Managing Feeder Cattle Health the First 30 Days on Feed

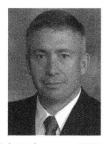 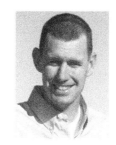

Daniel U. Thomson, DVM, PhD   Brad J. White, DVM, MS
Editors

Beef cattle health and well-being are important to providing a safe, wholesome beef product to the dinner table of the beef consumer. While feedlot cattle health can be influenced by many aspects outside the control of the farmer, rancher, and veterinarian, we must strive to develop practices that prevent disease occurrence and enhance cattle treatment outcomes. The two reasons cattle get sick are an overwhelming dose of a pathogen, a suppressed immune system, or a combination of the two. From the time the cattle step off the truck until they are moved onto the finish ration in their home pen, there are many health management practices that can be employed to minimize cattle stress and improve cattle health.

This publication has brought feedlot experts across the United States and Canada together to discuss the management of feedlot cattle health. It is important to understand the difference cattle management prior to arrival can make on health outcomes and prearrival management related to tailoring animal health programs at the feedlot. Veterinarians need to consider the animals (age, prior management, commingling), management (labor, nutrition, pen space), weather or climate, animal behavior and outcomes (food safety, antibiotic residue avoidance, animal well-being), and much more when developing herd health and individual animal programs. A large focus of this publication discusses how to develop protocols and manage cattle through the feedlot production phase.

The pendulum of food animal veterinary medicine continues to swing from population to individual animal solutions, and then back again. The population is representative of the collective individuals. However, the issues surrounding food animal production can be influenced by the geographical region to the farm to the pen to the individual animal. All levels are important factors in decision-making for a veterinarian. Nutrition and cattle comfort are managed in a group (pen) setting, but individual animals succumb to metabolic and environmental conditions.

Vet Clin Food Anim 31 (2015) xi–xii
http://dx.doi.org/10.1016/j.cvfa.2015.05.001
0749-0720/15/$ – see front matter © 2015 Elsevier Inc. All rights reserved.

vetfood.theclinics.com

Keeping cattle healthy, providing a safe and secure beef supply, and sustaining our natural resources are important aspects to a sustainable beef production system. Beef cattle health and well-being are a cornerstone to all beef operations. We hope this issue of the *Veterinary Clinics of North America: Food Animal Practice* serves the beef cattle veterinarians, ranchers, and feedlot operators in their business.

Daniel U. Thomson, DVM, PhD
Department of Diagnostic Medicine
and Pathobiology
College of Veterinary Medicine
Kansas State University
1800 Denison Avenue
Manhattan, KS 66506, USA

Brad J. White, DVM, MS
Department of Clinical Sciences
College of Veterinary Medicine
Kansas State University
1800 Denison Avenue
Manhattan, KS 66506, USA

E-mail addresses:
dthomson@vet.k-state.edu (D.U. Thomson)
bwhite@vet.k-state.edu (B.J. White)

Feedlot Vaccination
Does It Really Matter?

Gerald Stokka, DVM, MS[a],*, Timothy J. Goldsmith, DVM, MPH[b]

KEYWORDS

- Vaccination • Immune response • Cattle • Populations • Prevention
- Revaccination • Protocols • Protection

KEY POINTS

- The proper application of vaccines to cattle populations requires knowledge of risk factors and production system factors to get optimum value for the population being addressed as well as for the producer.
- By following the principles of a vaccination strategy as to necessity, efficacy, and safety, vaccine use and expectations become realistic.
- Veterinarians are qualified to make informed recommendations regarding cattle sourcing, animal handling, personnel training, judicious antimicrobial use, specific vaccine type, the timing of boosters, and the frequency of vaccination.

INTRODUCTION

The practice of vaccination to produce an immune response has been used to reduce the risk of infectious disease for more than 200 years.[1] Regarding the health of livestock, vaccination remains one of the most important management tools for the prevention of infectious disease. As such, it is imperative that veterinarians are involved in the recommendation of the administration and use of efficacious vaccines, resulting in the desired protective immune response.

The history of vaccine development and administration is replete with evidence of successful efforts to control both human and livestock pathogens. There are also numerous observations and evidence of the failure of vaccines and vaccinations to prevent transmission, infection, and clinical manifestations of disease caused by various pathogens. Although vaccines have been used commercially for more than 70 years, they have not changed greatly. They are still mostly the products of either live or killed whole virus or bacterial culture. However, the development of technology

Disclosure: The authors have nothing to disclose.
[a] Department of Animal Sciences, North Dakota State University, Hultz Hall, 1300 Albrecht Ave, Fargo, ND 58102, USA; [b] Center for Animal Health and Food Safety, College of Veterinary Medicine, University of Minnesota, 1365 Gortner Ave, Minneapolis, MN 55108, USA
* Corresponding author.
E-mail address: gerald.stokka@ndsu.edu

related to adjuvants, protective epitope identification, marker vaccines, and delivery systems is very active.

IMMUNIZATION VERSUS VACCINATION

The term vaccination comes from the Latin term vaccinus, which means of or from the cow. The relationship of this term to vaccination results from the efforts to prevent smallpox in the human population. It was determined that people with contact with cows with demonstrable lesions caused by the cowpox virus were significantly less likely to contract the highly contagious and serious human disease known as small-pox.[2] Vaccination therefore refers to the act or procedure of administering a vaccine.

There are several responses that can occur following the administration of a vaccine. The animal may not respond in any measurable way to the administered vaccine, or may have a weak measurable response. Alternatively, the animal may respond with a multitude of immune effects. The immune response may be beneficial to the animal in terms of protection against a specific pathogen or the immune response may result in an enhanced immune response that results in increased disorder of the target organ.[3] Thus it is presumptuous to assume that the administration of a vaccine to an individual or a population of animals results in immunization or protection.

PHILOSOPHY OF VACCINATION

The rationale of preventing infectious disease through planned vaccination strategies is critical to practicing veterinarians. Vaccination strategies should be well thought out, researched, and subject to continual review. Three principles should be considered when implementing vaccination protocols.

1. Necessary: is the risk of exposure high enough that clinical disease and pathogen transmission will become a health and well-being issue beyond the expectations for the group?
2. Efficacy: is there scientific evidence or observational experience that vaccine selection for specific pathogens is effective for the level of exposure and stress of the group?
3. Safety: is there evidence that vaccination will not cause harm, either through local or systemic reactions?

The result of considering these principles is that vaccination protocols become short, can be defended, and vaccines are used in the proper circumstances at the proper time. For example, on high-risk calves entering a backgrounding facility, only those products that are necessary to promote the respiratory health and well-being of the group should be used. A modified live viral respiratory vaccine may be the main product used in this situation.

VACCINATION AND POPULATION DYNAMICS

Methods to control disease in beef cattle populations have traditionally been focused on immunization to prevent clinical disease. Although prevention or reduction of the severity of clinical disease can be a direct effect of immunization, the indirect effect of disease prevention by decreasing pathogen transmission is of primary importance with pathogens that are transmitted from animal to animal.[4]

The concept of population/herd immunity has successfully been used to implement vaccination programs designed to protect human populations against disease pathogens. Specifically, they include diphtheria, tetanus, and pertussis; also measles, mumps, and rubella; as well as poliomyelitis.[5] Although there is concern about each individual being protected against disease, the greater purpose is to immunize as many individuals as possible within the population such that susceptible individuals within a population are also protected. A greater level of population protection can be achieved by:

1. Reducing the number of individuals shedding disease pathogens
2. Decreasing the amount of pathogen shed by infected individuals
3. Decreasing the duration of pathogen shedding
4. Increasing the pathogen infectious dose necessary to cause infection

In a confined cattle environment, a level of immunity in the population is necessary to reduce health risk to animals that are susceptible or at least partially susceptible to infection and its consequences. At the individual animal level, infection with a specific virus or bacterium is likely to occur regardless of immune status. With infection comes replication and spread to other target organs. This replication phase most often results in some degree of shedding the organism via nasal secretions, urine, feces, saliva, or ocular fluids. This replication leads to immune and inflammatory responses and produces signs and symptoms related to behavior and the effect on the primary target organ in the infected animal. Individual and population immunity can serve to short circuit this infectious process in several ways. Again, at the individual animal level, the immune response decreases the load of pathogens that is shed by infected animals and also the duration or length of shedding of infected animals. Within a population of immune animals, both of these pathogen reduction objectives are achieved. Thus, the efficiency of transmission is reduced individually and collectively and the number of animals shedding is reduced. Ultimately, the pathogen is unable to continue to be transmitted and infect susceptible individuals, with the eventual result of halting the spread and consequences of the pathogen.

The percentage of immune individuals in a population that is needed to achieve herd protection varies by disease pathogen, but ranges from 83% to 94%.[6] This concept is the basic premise of herd vaccination programs. The spread of pathogens within a population depends on the basic reproductive rate (R_o) of the specific pathogen.[7] The basic reproduction number R_o is the number of secondary infections resulting from 1 primary case in a susceptible population. R_o is a feature of both the infectious agent and the host population without a control measure being active. If R_o in a vaccinated population is larger than 1, then the vaccine cannot totally prevent the spread of infection and additional biosecurity principles must be used.[8] It has been estimated that for bovine herpes virus type 1 (BHV-1) infections the R_o is approximately 7.0. After using 2 different vaccines it was estimated that R_o was 2.4 and 1.1.[9] This means that, within these immunized populations, 2.4 and or 1.1 new cases will arise from 1 case. In this citation, population transmission could not effectively be prevented. Within real populations these numbers must be considered within the context that, as animals become infected and are contagious, the number of susceptible animals declines and the number of recovered and immune animals increases.

The critical proportion of immune animals needed to prevent transmission is expressed by the equation: critical proportion = $1 - 1/R_o$. The higher the R_o the greater the number of animals that must be immune in order to prevent spread of the infectious agent. If $R_o = 7.0$ for a specific pathogen, then the proportion of immune animals within that population must be $1 - (1/7)$, which means that approximately 86% of the population must be immune in order to prevent transmission. Estimates for limiting the spread of bovine virus diarrhea virus (BVDV) within a population have been made based on mathematical models.[10] In herds without persistently infected animals (PIs), 57% of the animals must be immune in order to stop transmission. For herds with PIs, 97% must be immune. The issue of herd immunity to BVDV is further complicated by the amount of cross-protection to the varied field strains afforded by commercial vaccines, and the desired level of protection. Protection against respiratory infection and clinical disease is reported to be less difficult to achieve than protecting the dam and developing fetus from infection.[11] In addition, vaccines must contain the major genotypes of field viruses in order to adequately prevent transmission by reducing the number of animals shedding virus and the amount of virus shedding by individual animals.[12] A sound recommendation for vaccines can only be made based on challenge models and field trials using good experimental design in applicable populations.

The challenge of making sound vaccination recommendations as part of an overall herd health program is the responsibility of food animal veterinarians. Making those recommendations requires an in-depth knowledge of the risk of disease, management ability, facilities, husbandry, and labor. In addition, veterinarians must have a working knowledge of the relative efficacy, duration of immunity, and the impact on transmission of the available commercial vaccines. Only recently has more of this type of information become available to practicing veterinarians.[13] With this as a working tool, veterinarians can use the concept of population dynamics and population immunity when making specific recommendations regarding the timing and frequency of vaccination administration.

CONCOMITANT ADMINISTRATION

In livestock production the practice of giving vaccines for multiple antigens either in combination or concurrently has become commonplace. Cattle production in specific geographic regions of the United States is characterized by a cow/calf sector that uses large areas of rangeland to raise and grow beef calves. Because of the extensive nature of production, beef calves may not be easily accessible to apply prevention or treatment protocols. The time between birth and weaning may only allow 1 or 2 working events. Thus, there is a need to administer multiple antigens at 1 event to conveniently and efficiently reduce the risk of common infectious diseases. The main focus of preventive health programs in young calves is the use of respiratory vaccines to stimulate protective immune responses. A common vaccination schedule for spring-born calves is to administer a viral respiratory vaccine along with a respiratory bacterial component either in a combination or given concurrently.[14] In addition to these, a multiple antigen clostridial vaccine is almost always administered.

Thus, preventive health vaccine strategies may include as many as 9 or 10 different antigens, given all at the same time. A question that deserves a response is whether all animals within a group are able to respond equally well to this number of antigens given at the same time or whether certain antigens interfere or negatively affect the response to other administered antigens.

Vaccines licensed and sold commercially throughout the Unites States are evaluated for efficacy and safety. When these criteria are met, a license for the vaccine label is issued. The wording of the label has some relationship with the prelicensing studies related to efficacy. The highest efficacy standard is labeled "Prevention of infection," the next lower standard "Prevention of disease," followed by "Aids in disease prevention," and "Aids in disease control."[15] When vaccines are given separately but concurrently, there is no obligation by manufacturers to communicate efficacy and safety standards. When vaccines are administered in combination, the standard for efficacy is that there is no demonstrable interference, which means that each antigenic fraction has met the efficacy and safety standards with no negative impact from other fractions.

The immune system has a defense mechanism that is ready at all times to respond to foreign antigens. The initial exposure to antigens may begin with an attempted invasion by breaching the innate immune system. The innate immune system is composed of many different mechanisms. The skin, a barrier that includes the epidermis and dermal layers, is virtually impenetrable unless there is an insult. Insults can be scratches, incisions, microscopic abrasions, burns, and even insect bites. The mucosal lining is also a barrier and part of the innate immune system; this barrier is more penetrable because the cells lining the mucosa are more absorptive and secretory. If these barriers have been breached, other mechanisms become involved. Immune cells in close proximity respond to invasion through tissue injury and toll-like receptors (TLRs). TLRs are located on the cells that line these barriers, and serve as sentries to alert the adaptive immune system that a foreign antigen has been detected.

In addition to TLRs, once a foreign antigen is encountered and phagocytosed by either macrophages or dendritic cells, an internal process is begun. This process involves specific select antigens that are then presented to helper T cells (Th1, Th2) via the major histocompatibility complex (MHC) receptors to direct the immune response. In naive animals the processing function is mainly driven by dendritic cells; these cells are able to present antigen via both MHC (1 and 2) receptor sites. These different receptor sites, along with Th1 and Th2 cells, result in the immune response being driven primarily toward a cell-mediated response, a humoral response, or both effector responses.

Several recent studies have shown biased and mixed Th1 and Th2 responses to bacterins, as shown by decreased antibody production to vaccination when concurrent or combination MLV/bacterin vaccines were administered.[16,17] Olajumoke and colleagues[18] showed a preferential Th1 response to pertussis vaccination in contrast with other pertussis vaccines, showing a preference for Th2 or a mixed Th1/Th2 response. In the case of pertussis in humans, it seems that the preferred Th1 primary response is the most protective.[19] Protection from intracellular bacterial infections such as *Mycoplasma bovis* also seem to require a primary Th1 response.[20] Viral infections and vaccines designed to elicit a protective immune response must also drive the Th1 response to protect and clear the infection. A response skewed toward a Th2 response can be detrimental, particularly with bovine respiratory syncytial virus (BRSV) infections.[21] An important consideration remains: does concomitant or concurrent administration elicit the appropriate immune response or does the response become biased by certain antigens contained in the vaccine combination or concurrently administered products? Challenge models designed to evaluate efficacy are the standard of vaccine production, but some vaccines are simply evaluated based on antibody responses to specific antigens that may or may not be protective.

LOGICAL VACCINATION PROTOCOLS

For veterinarians in food animal practice there are questions as to efficacy, duration of immunity, and number of doses needed to achieve a significant level of population and individual animal protection.[22,23] Veterinarians are called on to make recommendations concerning vaccination protocols for multiple diverse livestock businesses. To do so they require in-depth herd knowledge regarding some assessment of risk for specific diseases, management, genetics, nutritional status, and handling facilities. In confined cattle operations when vaccination programs are specifically outlined, it is uncommon for buyers to seek veterinary advice as to the quality of the program.

In BHV-1 vaccinated animals, some level of protective immunity against clinical diseases is assumed regardless of the type of vaccine. However, published comparisons between types of vaccines suggest a clear advantage, with modified live vaccines providing superior clinical disease and herd protection.[24–26]

Although the issue of safety, convenience, duration of immunity, and herd protection may be debated, perhaps the larger issue for veterinarians is that of risk analysis and risk management. What is the risk of the herd, group, or population being exposed to a field challenge with either infectious bovine rhinotracheitis (IBR) or bovine virus diarrhea virus (BVDV)? For confined cattle operations, this risk is assumed, and centers on the control of animal movements.[27] With stocker and feedlot cattle operations, this becomes more difficult, in that the source of incoming cattle and the level and stress of commingling before and on arrival result in exposure being likely. However, in a business with a system in place for disease control, the veterinarian is likely to recommend methods to both lower the risk of exposure and increase specific immunity to the pathogens considered to be of greatest risk. For example, reducing the exposure risk to common calf diarrhea pathogens has provided positive results when applied to calving systems.[28] This management also has a place in confined cattle operations. Pen size, grass traps, stocking rate, and pen density are all terms that should be part of the veterinarian management vocabulary. Increasing space or decreasing animal density within pen or grass traps decreases the number of contact possibilities between animals. In most cases, contact will eventually occur, but slowing the rate of exposure to commingled animals gives susceptible animals the opportunity to respond to vaccination procedures as well as overcoming the initial stressors associated with shipping; handling; processing; and, most importantly, commingling.

At present, calf health and weaning programs emphasize specific bovine respiratory disease (BRD) vaccination protocols and weaning for at least 45 days. Is 45 days a magic number that eliminates most of the BRD complex (BRDC) risk associated with weaning, or does it have some basis in science? The number of days before marketing calves after weaning has been arrived at by trial and error (mostly error). Some of the first weaning and vaccination programs to promote sales of weaned calves included weaning for a minimum of 21 days.[29] This period was soon increased to a minimum of 30 days and then increased again to 45 days.[30]

The principles of population dynamics and herd immunity are essential to understanding this time frame. In a group of 100 calves, with the stress of weaning, sorting, and handling all occurring at a single point in time, and weaned calves commingled from several pastures, it may be possible to predict the time to build herd immunity in most weaned calf groups. Assuming little shedding of pathogens before day 5, incubation periods on average of 5 days, and the force of the pathogen exposure from a single calf (excluding viral exposure) to be 3 (reproductive rate), then by day 10 3 more calves would be shedding and perhaps experiencing some signs or symptoms of BRD, assuming a constant contact rate. The assumption of a constant contact rate is unlikely, depending on pen space and animal movements, and therefore in most cases the spread is slower, especially with less contagious pathogens. Some of these exposures never result in clinical cases, but shedding still occurs. By day 45, this mild outbreak has progressed through the group, the impact of the stress of weaning is over, and the calves are at a greatly reduced risk of BRD.

In a review of literature, Taylor[31] implied economic reasons to the cow calf producer as the reason for the increased minimum number of days weaned. The economic logic was that the decreasing cost of gain and improvements in gain with increasing the number of days in the preconditioning period were the incentive for longer weaning periods.[31] Although this can be true with proper husbandry and nutrition, the value of weaned and conditioned calves began to change when the cost of illness became more accurately quantified.[32] The value of preconditioned calves is ultimately determined by the marketplace. The value is a function of the reputation of the cattle, regarding husbandry, genetics, nutrition, and health.[33] The main driver in weaned and conditioned calves has been health. Although vaccination is an important component of providing healthy calves to the marketplace, it is clear that the process of weaning and the amount of time after weaning and before sale is critical to reducing the risk of BRD. The belief used to be that vaccination was one of the primary determinants of the health of weaned calves, but little evidence exists to make that claim. Step and colleagues[14] found minimal differences in postweaning health with preconditioned (weaned [45 days] and vaccinated) calves compared with nonvaccinated weaned (45 days) calves. However, there may be beneficial indirect population effects of vaccination that influence the number of immune animals within a herd, resulting in reducing the spread of pathogen transmission within a herd and ultimately resulting in the infection dying out or becoming extinct.[34] However, in the case of BRDC in newly arrived calves in the feedlot, the positive impact of vaccination inducing herd immunity seems to be more difficult to show.[35] As a result, arrival programs for calves (particularly high and ultra–high risk) should include recommendations for low-stress handling, animal spacing, sanitation of processing and treatment areas, palatable receiving diets, and prophylactic antibiotic use.

REVACCINATION

The concept and the term revaccination are used in contrast with booster vaccination. Revaccination in the population sense is the administering of a second vaccine to a population such that a greater percentage of the population has the opportunity to produce a protective immune response. Booster vaccination implies that the second vaccination will boost or improve the immune response following the initial or primary dose. The literature supporting the use of revaccination is limited and does not show a positive benefit in most cases.[36] The logic for the use of revaccination is that calves on arrival at a new facility with concomitant stress will have fewer individuals responding to an initial dose of vaccine. Typically a second dose in a revaccination protocol is given between 7 and 14 days following the initial dose. This second dose provides those individuals not responding initially with the opportunity to respond immunologically, following rest, water intake, and feed consumption. The rationale is that, in confined, stressed new cattle, there is a sensitive period of time to build immunity and protection before infection and clinical signs become evident in most of the population. In a population of calves there may be 3 responses to revaccination. The calves that responded to the initial dose on arrival do not respond to the second dose, calves not responding initially have the opportunity to respond, and some calves on receiving either the initial dose or the revaccination dose may develop an anamnestic or booster response if they had been exposed or vaccinated before arrival. Typically, revaccination protocols are only used with the modified live respiratory virus vaccines. There has been some concern that, if there is continued stress and pathogen exposure, revaccination may aggravate an already tenuous health status in groups of calves. Stokka and Edwards[37] showed no negative effects of multiple revaccinations in highly stressed calves. Revaccination strategies and the parameters for their use are the responsibility of practicing veterinarians. Not every group requires revaccination within 7 to 14 days period because it depends on sourcing; previous group history; and, at times, environmental conditions. In specific circumstances, such as unexpected rates of BRD occurring later in the receiving phase, revaccination has also been used.

REASONABLE EXPECTATIONS

The expectations that come with the use of vaccines have been, and will continue to be, unrealistic. Even the most efficacious vaccine on the market, with an efficacy of 90% against clinical disease, shedding, and transmission when used in challenge models on healthy animals, will be considerably compromised when used in stressed, commingled animals of unknown health and history.

What is the appropriate expectation for response rates to vaccination under field conditions? For disease challenges other than BRD, the expectations seem to be more predictable. The disease challenge associated with the clostridial (blackleg) species and protection through vaccination seem to highly effective. A 1923 Agricultural Experiment Station bulletin from the Kansas State Agricultural College cites 10% to 20% losses associated with blackleg, whereas vaccination reduced losses to less than 1%.[38]

Results such as these may have created unrealistic expectations for the use of respiratory vaccines. In cattle in the feedlot, the predominant respiratory disease event is associated with BRDC. The term complex implies that clinical respiratory disease is more than the simple presence of bacteria resulting in infection and clinical disease; it is the result of a multitude of risk factors combining with infectious pathogens. The predominant bacteria associated with respiratory disease in cattle, such as *Mannheimia haemolytica*, *Pasteurella haemolytica*, and *Histophilus somni* are commonly found in the nasopharyngeal passage in healthy normal cattle. The transmission of these organisms in the population is not well understood, but they seem to be only moderately transmissible even with pathogenic species.[39] In contrast, *M bovis* seems to be highly contagious, may maintain a persistent state in infected animals, and can rapidly spread in susceptible populations.[40] The main immune response elicited by killed bacterin vaccines is the humoral response, which is primarily one of building antibody to the protective epitopes identified and processed by components of the immune system. With *M haemolytica*, antibody production for the leukotoxin of the organism has been well shown to reduce lung lesions; however, other antibody responses are necessary to prevent excessive multiplication and infection in lung tissue.[41] Protective antibodies induced by vaccination with *Pasteurella* and *Histophilus* species seem to be less effective and understood.[42] The respiratory bacterin vaccines seem to be most effective when placed well before exposure and stress. Antibody is the slowest immune response elicited by the immune system.[43–45] Thus, the opportunity for protection early after arrival is limited unless previous exposure has occurred.

Expectations for the viral respiratory vaccines are different. Vaccination is the only tool to effectively manage viral infectious agents. Brock and colleagues[46] showed that onset of at least partial protection against BVDV could be as early as 3 days after modified live vaccination. Viral pathogens depend on intracellular machinery for multiplication and spread, which means that the cell-mediated response is the critical immune response to provide protection. Antibody production is induced as well, which serves to help limit viremia and transmission. The category of modified live vaccines has been shown to be the most effective at producing this type of protective response. At present, most commercial products contain BHV-1, Parinfluenza 3 virus (PI3V), BRSV, and type 1 and 2 BVDV fractions. Whether all of these agents are necessary for all regions of the country is open to debate, but the BHV-1 and BVDV fractions have been shown to be necessary and effective.[45] Recently, increased interest has resulted in more vaccines becoming available that require intranasal administration. It is clear that, for some of the respiratory pathogens, particularly BRSV, protection is provided by this delivery method. Because this site is the natural route of exposure, and at the mucosal surface immunoglobulin A is the predominant protective antibody, it is logical that vaccination at this site is superior to the parenteral route of administration.[47] In addition, the induced memory response provides feedback to the site of administration even when conventional vaccines are given as the booster dose.[48] It is clear that the respiratory viral vaccines are effective against specific viruses that are implicated in the BRDC.

RECOMMENDATIONS

The goal of any prevention program is to reduce the risks associated with the development of clinical disease. By following the principles of a vaccination strategy regarding necessity, efficacy, and safety, vaccine use and expectations become realistic. In high-risk calves, use only what is necessary to promote health and well-being. For the BRDC, clinicians too often reduce only the risk associated with the infectious component. Other risk factors often overcome the beneficial effects of an immune response, and as a result clinicians are often disappointed in the results. In moderate-risk to low-risk calves, less may be better because the major contributors to the BRDC have been ameliorated. Veterinarians perform a vital service in this way and are qualified to make informed recommendations regarding cattle sourcing, animal handling, personnel training, judicious antimicrobial use, specific vaccine type, the timing of boosters, and the frequency of vaccination.

REFERENCES

1. Lombard M, Pastoret PP, Moulin AM. A brief history of vaccines and vaccination. Rev Sci Tech 2007;26(1):29–48.
2. Abbas K. Cellular and molecular immunology. 5th edition. Philadelphia: Saunders; 2003. ISBN 0-7216-0008-5.
3. Slocombe RF, Malark J, Ingersoll R, et al. Importance of neutrophils in the pathogenesis of acute pneumonic pasteurellosis in calves. Am J Vet Res 1985;46: 2253–8.
4. Halloran ME, Haber M, Longini IM, et al. Direct and indirect effects in vaccine efficacy and effectiveness. Am J Epidemiol 1991;133(4):323–31.
5. Anderson RM. The concept of herd immunity and the design of community-based immunization programmes. Vaccine 1992;10(13):928–35.
6. May T, Silverman RD. 'Clustering of exemptions' as a collective action threat to herd immunity. Vaccine 2003;21(11–12):1048–51.
7. Stokka GL. Population dynamics and herd immunity. In: Proceedings of the 41st Annual Conference of the AABP. Stillwater (OK): VM Publishers; 2008.
8. Noordhuizen JP, Frankena K, van der Hoofd CM, et al. Application of quantitative methods in veterinary epidemiology. Wageningen (The Netherlands): Wageningen Pers; 1997. p. 249–69.
9. Bosch JC. Bovine herpesvirus 1 marker vaccines: tools for eradication? [PhD thesis] Utrech, The Netherlands: University of Utrecht; 1997.
10. Cherry BR, Reeves MJ, Smith G. Evaluation of bovine viral diarrhea virus control using a mathematical model of infection dynamics. Prev Vet Med 1998;33: 91–108.
11. Ficken MD, Ellsworth MA, Tucker CM, et al. Effects of modified-live bovine viral diarrhea virus vaccines containing either type 1 or types 1 and 2 BVDV on heifers and their offspring after challenge with noncytopathic type 2 BVDV during gestation. J Am Vet Med Assoc 2006;228(10):1559–64.

12. Thurmond MC. Virus transmission. In: Goyal SM, Ridpath JF, editors. Bovine viral diarrhea virus: diagnosis management and control. Oxford (United Kingdom): Blackwell Publishing; 2005. p. 91–104.

13. Newcomer BW, Walz PH, Givens MD, et al. Efficacy of bovine viral diarrhea virus vaccination to prevent reproductive disease: a meta-analysis. Theriogenology 2015;83:360–5.

14. Step DL, Krehbiel CR, DePra HA, et al. Effects of commingling beef calves from different sources and weaning protocols during a forty-two-day receiving period on performance and bovine respiratory disease. J Anim Sci 2008;86(11):3146–58.

15. Veterinary Services Memorandum No. 800.202. Available at: http://www.aphis. usda.gov/animal_health/vet_biologics/publications/memo_800_202.pdf.

16. Cortese VS, Seeger JT, Stokka GL, et al. Serological response to *Mannheimia haemolytica* in calves concurrently administered inactivated or modified live preparations of *M. haemolytica* and viral combination vaccines containing modified live bovine herpesvirus type 1. Am J Vet Res 2011;72(11):1541–9.

17. Stoltenow C, Cortese JT, Seeger GL, et al. Immunologic responses of beef calves to concurrent application of modified-live viral vaccine (intranasal and systemic administration) and systemically administered *Mannheimia haemolytica* bacterin-leukotoxoid. Bovine Pract 2011;45(2):132–9.

18. Fadugba OO, Wang L, Chen Q, et al. Immune responses to pertussis antigens in infants and toddlers after immunization with multicomponent acellular pertussis vaccine. Clin Vaccine Immunol 2014;21(12):1613–9.

19. Mascart F, Berscheure V, Malfroot A, et al. *Bordatella pertussis* infection in 2-month-old infants promotes type 1 T cell responses. J Immunol 2003;170: 1504–9.

20. Mulongo M, Prysliak T, Perez-Casal J. Vaccination of feedlot cattle with extracts and membrane fractions from two *Mycoplasma bovis* isolates results in strong humoral immune responses but does not protect against an experimental challenge. Vaccine 2013;31:1406–12.

21. Gershwin LJ. Immunology of bovine respiratory syncytial virus infection of cattle. Comp Immunol Microbiol Infect Dis 2012;35:253–7.

22. Ellis J, Walden C, Ricketts V. Longevity of protective immunity to experimental bovine herpes-1 infection following inoculation with a combination modified-live virus vaccine in beef calves. J Am Vet Med Assoc 2005;227(1):123–8.

23. Fulton RW, Johnson BJ, Briggs RE, et al. Challenge with bovine viral diarrhea virus by exposure to persistently infected calves: protection by vaccination and negative results of antigen testing in nonvaccinated acutely infected calves. Can J Vet Res 2006;70:121–7.

24. Rodning SP, Marley MS, Zhang Y, et al. Comparison of three commercial vaccines for preventing persistent infection with bovine viral diarrhea virus. Theriogenology 2010;73(8):1154–63.

25. Bosch JC, Kaashoek MJ, Kroese AH, et al. An attenuated bovine herpesvirus 1 marker vaccine induces a better protection than two inactivated marker vaccines. Vet Microbiol 1996;52:223–34.

26. Castrucci G, Frigeri F, Salvatori D, et al. Vaccination of calves against bovine herpesvirus-1: assessment of the protective value of eight vaccines. Comp Immunol Microbiol Infect Dis 2002;25:29–41.

27. Ezanno P, Fourichon C, Beaudeau F, et al. Between-herd movements of cattle as a tool for evaluating the risk of introducing infected animals. Anim Res 2006; 55(3):189–208.

28. Smith DR, Grotelueshen D, Knott T, et al. Managing to alleviate calf scours: the Sandhills calving system. In: Proceedings, The Range Beef Cow Symposium XVIII. Mitchell (NE): VM Publishers; 2003.
29. Wieringa FL, Curtis RA, Willoughby RA. The influence of preconditioning on plasma corticosteroid levels, rectal temperatures and the incidence of shipping fever in beef calves. Can Vet J 1976;17:280–6.
30. Schipper C, Church T, Harris B. A review of the Alberta certified preconditioned feeder program – 1980–1987. Can Vet J 1989;30:736–40.
31. Taylor AM. The effect of castration timing and preconditioning program on beef calf performance [MS Thesis]. Gainesville (FL): University of Florida; 2011.
32. 1999–2000 Texas A&M Ranch to Rail - North/South Summary. Available at: animalscience.tamu.edu/wp-content/uploads/.../beef-r2r-992000.pdf. Accessed April 14, 2012.
33. Zimmerman LC, Schroeder TC, Dhuyvetter KC, et al. The effect of value-added management on calf prices at superior livestock auction video markets. J Agr Resource 2012;37(1):128–43.
34. De Jong CM, Bouma A. Herd immunity after vaccination: how to quantify it and how to use it to halt disease. Vaccine 2001;19:2722–8.
35. Windeyer MC, Leslie KE, Godden SM, et al. The effects of viral vaccination of dairy heifer calves on the incidence of respiratory disease, mortality, and growth. J Dairy Sci 2012;95(11):6731–9.
36. Step DL, Krehbiel CR, Burciaga-Robles LO, et al. Comparison of single vaccination versus revaccination with a modified live virus vaccine containing bovine herpesvirus-1, bovine viral diarrhea virus (types 1a and 2a), parainfluenza type 3 virus, and bovine respiratory syncytial virus in the prevention of bovine respiratory disease in cattle. J Am Vet Med Assoc 2009;235(5):580–7.
37. Stokka GL, Edwards AJ. Revaccination of stressed calves with a multiple polyvalent MLV vaccine (IBR, BVD, PI3, BRSV). Agri Practice 1990;11(5):18–20.
38. Agricultural Experiment Station, Kansas State Agricultural College. Blackleg vaccines: their production and use. Topeka (KS): Kansas State Printing Plant; 1923. p. 9–5555 Technical Bulletin 10.
39. Timsit E, Christensen H, Bareille H, et al. Transmission dynamics of *Mannheimia haemolytica* in newly-received beef bulls at fattening operations. Vet Microbiol 2013;161:295–304.
40. Timsit E, Arcangioli MA, Bareille N, et al. Transmission dynamics of *Mycoplasma bovis* in newly received beef bulls at fattening operations. J Vet Diagn Invest 2012;24(6):1172–6.
41. Mosier DA, Panciera RJ, Rogers DP, et al. Comparison of serologic and protective responses induced by two *Pasteurella* vaccines. Can J Vet Res 1998;62(3):178–82.
42. Larson RL, Step DL. Evidence-based effectiveness of vaccination against *Mannheimia haemolytica*, *Pasteurella multocida*, and *Histophilus somni* in feedlot cattle for mitigating the incidence and effect of bovine respiratory disease complex. Vet Clin North Am Food Anim Pract 2012;28(1):97–106.
43. Babiuk LA, van Drunen Littel-van den Hurk S, Tikoo SK. Immunology of bovine herpesvirus 1 infection. Vet Microbiol 1996;53(1–2):31–42.
44. Palomares RA, Marley SM, Givens MD, et al. Bovine viral diarrhea virus fetal persistent infection after immunization with a contaminated modified-live virus vaccine. Theriogenology 2013;79(8):1184–95.

45. Theurer ME, Larson RL, White BJ. Systematic review and meta-analysis of the effectiveness of commercially available vaccines against bovine herpesvirus, bovine viral diarrhea virus, bovine respiratory syncytial virus, and parainfluenza type 3 virus for mitigation of bovine respiratory disease complex in cattle. J Am Vet Med Assoc 2015;246(1):126–42.

46. Brock KV, Widel P, Walz P, et al. Onset of protection from experimental infection with type 2 bovine viral diarrhea virus following vaccination with a modified-live vaccine. Vet Ther 2007;8(1):88–96.

47. Ellis J, Gow S, West K, et al. Response of calves to challenge exposure with virulent bovine respiratory syncytial virus following intranasal administration of vaccines formulated for parenteral administration. J Am Vet Med Assoc 2007; 230(2):233–43.

48. Shewen PE, Carrasco-Medina L, McBey BA, et al. Challenges in mucosal vaccination of cattle. Vet Immunol Immunopathol 2009;128(1–3):192–8.

Management of Preconditioned Calves and Impacts of Preconditioning

W. Mark Hilton, DVM

KEYWORDS

- Economics • Marketing • Preconditioning • Vaccination • Weaning

KEY POINTS

- Preconditioning (PC) calves can be an economically sound endeavor for the cow-calf producer.
- Focusing on factors such as weight gain, cost of gain, length of PC period, and marketing options that are under the control of the producer has been proved to increase profitability in producing PC calves.
- PC calves tend to sell at a higher price per hundredweight (cwt) than non-PC calves of similar weight and quality primarily because of a health sales price advantage.
- Demand for PC calves continues to grow even as the price per cwt increases.
- Compared with non-PC calves, PC calves have improved health, gain, feed efficiency, and animal welfare in the feedlot along with increased carcass weight and quality grade at slaughter.

INTRODUCTION

The concept of PC calves before sale was conceived in the mid-1960s by Iowa State University extension veterinarian Dr John Herrick (Hartwig N., personal communication, Iowa State University, 2010).[1] The goal was to decrease morbidity and mortality in the backgrounding lot or feedlot by marketing a calf that was vaccinated, castrated, dehorned, dewormed, weaned, and trained to eat from a bunk and drink from a water tank. In 1967, the Oklahoma State University hosted a national conference to discuss PC.[2] Some skepticism was evident when the process was initially described, but by the mid-1970s about 600,000 calves were PC in Iowa.[1,3]

Some of the earliest studies on PC showed that the process produced little to no return on investment to the cow-calf producer.[4,5] These studies from the 1960s to the mid-1980s used nutrition, genetics, technology, and health practices that were

The author has nothing to disclose.
Department of Veterinary Clinical Sciences, Purdue University College of Veterinary Medicine, 625 Harrison Street, West Lafayette, IN 47907, USA
E-mail address: hiltonw@purdue.edu

Vet Clin Food Anim 31 (2015) 197–207
http://dx.doi.org/10.1016/j.cvfa.2015.03.002
vetfood.theclinics.com

current for those times. Nearly 50 years later, there have been substantial improvements in each area, and PC must be examined with twenty-first century information and technology.

Benefits of Preconditioning for the Cow-Calf Producer

Numerous studies have demonstrated that the concept of PC is sound in the health production sense, but the economics of the program for the cow-calf producer and the feedlot owner have often been questioned.[6–10] Potential benefits of selling PC calves include selling additional weight, garnering a higher market price, and maintaining healthier calves.

Reduced shrink in preconditioning calves

All cattle incur shrink from the time cattle leave the farm or ranch of origin until delivery to the auction market or directly to the buyer. Unweaned calves typically shrink more than PC calves, and in a study by Barnes and colleagues,[11] 3 groups of calves were compared to measure shrink. Group 1 had been weaned 22 days before sale (not actually PC because of weaning for <30 days), group 2 was weaned the day of the sale, and group 3 was weaned the day before the sale. Shrink was 2.3% in the weaned calves, 3.4% in the just weaned calves, and 4.9% in the calves weaned the day before the sale. Although PC can decrease shrink, many studies conclude that the amount of stress in handling the cattle on the day of transport is an even more significant factor.[12] In the spreadsheet provided below (**Table 1**), a shrink of 2.3% is used on the PC calves and 3.4% is used on unweaned calves that were sold.

Selling additional weight

Most studies that examined the economic viability of PC focused primarily on the PC health sales price advantage (sometimes called the PC bonus) that was paid for these calves when compared with that paid for calves with no history.[6–8] Although this factor should garner some attention, the price paid is not under the control of the seller. Conversely, the pounds of calf sold is primarily under the control of the seller. The addition of pounds of salable weight to a calf at a cost of gain that is below the marginal return adds value to the calf and profit to the producer. Generally speaking, lighter calves have more efficient weight gain when compared with heavier calves, so the efficient time to add weight is to the young, newly weaned calf weighing 400 to 600 lb. The improved efficiency is because lighter calves use less energy for maintenance than heavier calves.

This efficiency of gain also leads to a reduced cost of gain when compared with heavier calves. Again, as calves get heavier, a greater quantity of calories are needed for maintenance functions. The calf owner receives payment for calf gain, not calf maintenance. Many studies or simulations of PC programs report calf gains of 1.0 to 1.5 lb/calf/d during a 45-day PC period.[6,8,9,13] Current studies show that gains of 3.0 lb/calf/d are attainable during this time frame.[14,15] In an 11-year study of a herd in Indiana, average daily gain (ADG) improved from 1.21 lb/calf/d the first year of the study to 2.87 lb/calf/d in year 5 and to 3.05 lb/calf/d by year 9.[14] As nutrition, genetics, and technology improved, so did ADG. It can also be argued that in addition to the nutritional aspect, PC calves seems to be a skill that improves with experience.

One of the keys to financial success in PC calves is improvement of gain of the calves.[14,16] In Donnell's[16] work at the Noble Foundation in Oklahoma in 2004–2005, the following conclusions were made based on commodity prices of that period and a 52-day PC period[16]:

- A 0.2-lb increase in ADG (or 10.4 lb in 52 days) produced a net profit of $4.25/ head.

Table 1
Impact of ADG on cost of gain and profitability in 2014

Feedstuff, lb/head/d	Ration #1	Ration #2	Ration #3
Dry distiller's grains with solubles (lb)	0	1.25	3
Cracked corn (lb)	0	2.75	6.5
Coproduct balancer with ionophore (lb)	0.5	0.5	0.5
Alfalfa/grass hay (lb)	15.2	12	6
ADG (lb)	1.0	2.0	3.0
Feed cost/head/d ($)	1.64	1.65	1.54
Feed cost/lb gain ($)	1.64	0.83	0.51
Feed:gain, dry matter (DM) basis	12.9:1	6.9:1	4.6:1
Weight at start of the PC program (lb)	500	500	500
Calf price ($/cwt)	296.80	296.80	296.80
% shrink if calf sold on the day of weaning	3.40	3.40	3.40
Weight with shrink (lb)	483	483	483
Calf value/head, day of weaning ($)	1433.54	1433.54	1433.54
Interest rate (%)	5	5	5
Labor cost @ $0.20/head/d ($)	9.00	9.00	9.00
Vaccinations, dewormer, implant ($)	13.60	13.60	13.60
Processing charge ($)	5.00	5.00	5.00
Feed cost ($)	73.80	74.25	69.30
Yardage cost @ $0.25/d ($)	11.25	11.25	11.25
Interest on calf, 5%, 45 days ($)	8.84	8.84	8.84
Death loss, 0.5% ($)	7.42	7.42	7.42
Total cost of program ($)	128.91	129.36	124.41
Cost/d in PC program ($)	2.86	2.87	2.76
Weight gained (lb)	45	90	135
Cost/lb of gain ($)	2.86	1.44	0.92
Days in PC program	45	45	45
Financial analysis			
Weight after PC (lb)	545	590	635
% shrink at sale	2.30	2.30	2.30
Weight at PC sale with shrink (lb)	532	576	620
Price per cwt at PC sale, no PC bonus included ($)	286.00	276.55	266.47
Value of PC calf at sale, no PC bonus included ($)	1522.85	1594.12	1653.17
Profit (loss) of PC, no PC bonus included ($)	(39.60)	31.22	95.22
Price per cwt at PC sale, $12.06 PC bonus included ($)	298.06	288.61	278.53
Value of PC calf at sale, PC bonus of $12.06/cwt included ($)	1624.43	1702.80	1768.67
Profit (loss) of PC, PC bonus of $12.06/cwt included ($)	61.98	139.90	210.71
% return on investment	48.1	108.1	169.4

Feed cost used ($/ton as fed basis): DDGS $120, corn $125, balancer $600, hay $150. Price slide is $22.50/cwt, which was typical for markets in fall 2014. All sale prices include shrink.
  (*Data from* www.mwbeefcattle.com.)

- Each $1 increase in feed/mineral cost reduced net margins by $1.47/head.
- Each $1 increase in hay cost reduced net margins by $2.31/head.

Prices in December 2004 and 2005 were as follows[17–19]:

- Corn: $1.93/bushel or $68.93/ton
- Alfalfa hay: $94.35/ton
- 500 to 550 lb calves: $88.99/cwt

Prices for 2014 are used in the example in **Table 1**, and although 2014 corn price is double the price in the 2004–2005 price, the price of hay is only marginally higher than that in 2004–2005. The largest price differential though is in calf price where the 2014 prices are 3.1 times higher than when Donnell[16] conducted her research. To demonstrate the impact of ADG on cost of gain and profitability in 2014, 3 separate rations that are fed to 500 lb steers over a 45-day PC period were formulated (see **Table 1**). The rations are fed at 100% projected intake and balanced to produce gains of 1.0 lb/d, 2.0 lb/d, or 3.0 lb/d over a 45-day period.

This partial budget analysis shows that improving ADG, in most cases, leads to increased profitability for the cow-calf producer. It is no surprise that as ADG increases, the cost of gain decreases. What is a surprise to many is that the feed cost per head per day actually decreases as the ADG increases. The cost per ton of energy on a dry matter basis is typically highest for rations that have an abundance of low-energy-dense feeds such as hay. To keep calves gaining at a very low rate (~ 1 lb/head/d) a large portion of the ration must consist of low-energy-dense feeds. The higher ADG rations and lower cost per kilogram of gain rations are typically those that contain proportionally increased amounts of high-energy-dense feeds such as corn and dried distillers grains with solubles (DDGS). In the above example with the calves gaining 3 lb/d, 46% of the additional profit realized by selling PC calves was because of selling additional pounds, while the PC health sales price advantage accounted for 54%. The profit that came from selling additional pounds in this example is lower than the results of the 11-year study in Indiana with over 1100 calves in which 63% of additional profit was because of weight gain.[14] The average PC health sales price advantage in the 11-year study was only $6.01/cwt when compared with $12.06 in the above example. The Indiana study does corroborate that increasing ADG is positively correlated to overall profitability, and improving the ADG, which is under the control of the producer, should be acknowledged as an important aspect of profitability of PC when discussing this management/marketing strategy with the cow-calf producer.

To compare the above example (see **Table 1**) with the earlier study done by Donnell,[16] increasing ADG by 0.2 lb/d with 2014 prices would return $13.40 to net profit. This value is 3.15 times the return seen in the 2004–2005 study, and the value of calves/cwt is 3.10 times higher than the prices received in 2004–2005. So, higher-priced calves with relatively similar feed prices makes increasing ADG even more important to PC profitability for the cow-calf producer.

Nutritional consultation

If a cow-calf producer has never PC calves, it can be assumed that developing a post-weaning ration may prove to be a challenge. If a beef nutritionist is available to assist with this endeavor, using this expertise is likely the best option. If this is not the case, other people such as a feed company employee, extension beef specialist, or a veterinarian may assist in the formulation of a balanced ration that achieves gains that allow the calves' genetics and health to be optimized. Many computer-based nutrition programs are available for use in formulating PC rations, and these can be a valuable asset in the PC process.

Adding days to the preconditioning period

Another way to add weight is to lengthen the PC period. Many PC programs have evolved to 45 days or more versus the original 30-day period. While an improvement in immunity is part of the reason for the increased days, calf weight gain is another reason. It is generally accepted that if calves are weaned and fed for some time before being sold, the first week after weaning produces the poorest gain when compared with the subsequent weeks postweaning. In a 30-day PC period, 1 week represents 23% of the entire PC period. If calves are fed for 45 or 60 days, 1 week is only 16% or 12% of the entire feeding period, respectively, and the first week reduces the impact on overall gain. As long as the total cost of gain is below the marginal value of gain, the cow-calf producer should examine owning and feeding the calves for additional days.

In the Noble Foundation study in 2004–2005, each additional day added to the PC program increased the net margins by approximately $1.00/head. With 2014 prices and 3 lb/d gain, approximately $2.75/d would be added to the net profit for each additional day in the PC program. A potential negative of feeding for an extended period is that as calves become heavier, there may be reduced marketing opportunities, so this factor must be examined.

In any discussion of feeding calves in a PC program the subject of getting calves too fleshy is likely to surface. In fact, many articles on PC caution about getting calves too fleshy. When data was analyzed on 84,319 feeder calves selling in approximately 8200 lots in Kansas and Missouri in 2008–2009, the discount for calves of fat condition was $0.86/cwt and it made up only 6.4% of all calves sold.[20] In a similar study in Arkansas with 105,542 calves in 52,401 lots, the discount for fleshy calves was $5.82/cwt with 2.9% of the calves classified as fleshy.[21] Avent and colleagues[6] examined 1249 lots of feeder calves where those deemed to be in fleshy condition sold for a $0.60/cwt discount. The mean weight in the study was 520 lb, so the fleshy discount was $3.12/calf; the discount for thin condition in the same study was $0.52/cwt or $2.70/calf. It is not inconceivable to think that some calves that were PC and sold as average condition might have been thin if sold 30 to 45 days earlier without PC. PC programs are selling high health calves, and having calves with a bit more flesh could be seen as just healthy instead of fleshy.

In the 11-year case study in Indiana with calves gaining up to 3.05 lb/d, none of the calves of over 1100 total PC were labeled as fleshy.[14] It seems from the numerous studies on this subject that the risk of having fleshy calves when nutrition and genetics are matched to produce gains of 3.0 lb/d is minimal and possibly even a dogma.

Marketing preconditioned calves

For several years, data have been collected by researchers examining results of calves sold through a video auction service.[22,23] Calves are classified in various certified vaccination programs with or without a calf weaning component. In this data set from 1994 to 2012, over 54,000 lots representing 6.5 million cattle have been recorded and evaluated with regard to vaccination and weaning.

From 1994 to 2010, the percentage of calves that qualified for the VAC 45 program (vaccinated twice for IBR-BVD-PI$_3$-BRSV, 7-way clostridial organisms, *Mannheimia haemolytica*, and/or *Pasteurella multocida* and weaned ≥45 days, PC) increased from 1.8% in 1994 to 29.2% in 2010, an overall 16-fold increase (**Table 2**). The VAC 34 program (single Infectious bovine rhinotracheitis, bovine virus diarrhea, parainfluenza 3, bovine respiratory syncytial virus [IBR-BVD-PI$_3$-BRSV] with no weaning requirement or prewean vaccinated) showed increases from 8.3% in 1994 to 52.3% in 2009, a 6-fold increase.

Compared with nonviral vaccinated calves, health sales price advantage (or price premium) for VAC 45 calves in 1994 and 1995 was $0.25 and $2.74/cwt, respectively,

Table 2
Number of sale lots by year and value-added health program for beef calves sold through Superior Livestock video auctions

		Value Added Health Program Administered to Sale Lots, % of Total			
		Not Certified[a]		Vaccinated	
				Not Weaned	Weaned
Year	Total Number of Lots in Data Analysis	Not Vaccinated	Vaccinated	Certified[b]	Certified[c]
1994	1930	88.3	—	8.3	1.8
1995	1576	43.7	38.6	12.4	3.2
1996	1793	34.0	33.9	27.7	4.5
1997	1902	29.8	33.2	23.1	4.5
1998	2410	18.0	26.5	21.3	5.0
1999	2600	17.7	32.8	30.3	6.9
2000	2406	18.0	47.0	26.0	9.0
2001	2414	14.2	29.4	43.4	12.9
2002	2439	10.2	30.0	44.5	15.3
2003	3150	6.3	20.1	47.5	20.7
2004	3431	5.3	14.3	48.5	25.4
2005	3584	3.2	11.6	53.0	24.2
2006	3517	2.9	9.6	47.8	24.5
2007	4091	2.7	7.5	48.8	26.7
2008	3741	1.8	6.7	51.4	26.3
2009	3806	1.2	4.2	52.3	28.8
2010	3742	2.2	4.1	29.9	29.2
2011	3416	1.4	4.1	28.0	29.0
2012	2868	1.2	2.9	27.5	27.2

[a] Calves in this category were vaccinated against one or more of the following viruses at some time between birth and the date of sale: IBR, BVD, PI₃, and BRSV.
[b] VAC 34. For certification requirements, see http://www.superiorlivestock.com/files/vac_programs.pdf.
[c] VAC 45. For certification requirements, see http://www.superiorlivestock.com/files/vac_programs.pdf.
Courtesy of David Lalman, PhD, Department of Animal Science, Oklahoma State University, Stillwater, OK.

whereas prices in 2012 reached a premium of $12.06/cwt (**Table 3**). For VAC 34 calves, price premium was $0.77 and $1.35/cwt in 1994 and 1995, respectively, and in 2012, this premium had risen to $6.72/cwt. Although marketing of both VAC 34 and VAC 45 calves increased dramatically during the 19-year period, the percentage of calves that were classified as nonviral vaccinated dropped from 88.3% of total marketing in 1994 to 1.2% in 2012.

As numbers of PC calves, and to a lesser extent prewean vaccinated calves, increased, the value of these calves increased. In most instances as supply increases, demand and price decrease. In this case, the price continued to increase and was most likely due to positive feedback on profitability of these value-added calves in the feedlot. As the reputation of these calves became known, demand increased.

Cow-calf producers have long expressed skepticism regarding the likelihood of achieving premiums for value-added management practices. It is not surprising that risk-averse producers facing uncertain returns would be hesitant to adopt

Table 3
Effect of value-added health programs on the price of beef calves sold through Superior Livestock video auctions

	Value-Added Health Program Administered to Sale Lots			
			Not Weaned	Weaned
	Not Vaccinated	Vaccinated	Vaccinated	Vaccinated
	Not Certified	Not Certified[a]	Certified[b]	Certified[c]
Year	Price ($/cwt)	Premium Over Nonvaccinated and Noncertified ($/cwt)		
1994	83.80	—	0.77	0.25
1995	67.79	0.70	1.35	2.47
1996	61.79	0.43	0.99	3.35
1997	91.26	0.72	1.61	3.89
1998	73.86	0.74	1.38	3.35
1999	85.92	0.96	1.17	3.33
2000	100.06	1.27	1.76	3.66
2001	95.28	1.23	2.21	4.06
2002	79.95	1.10	1.80	5.01
2003	93.80	1.85	3.39	6.69
2004	116.05	1.71	3.47	7.91
2005	114.08	1.43	2.45	6.64
2006	119.96	1.92	3.41	7.61
2007	112.15	2.20	4.68	7.83
2008	104.90	2.19	3.57	8.20
2009	95.22	0.69	2.93	7.21
2010	112.28	1.15	3.02	6.14
2011	131.08	4.57	6.55	11.88
2012	152.30	5.26	6.72	12.06

[a] Calves in this category were vaccinated against one or more of the following viruses at some time between birth and the date of sale: IBR, BVD, PI_3, and BRSV.
[b] VAC 34. For certification requirements see http://www.superiorlivestock.com/files/vac_programs.pdf.
[c] VAC 45. For certification requirements see http://www.superiorlivestock.com/files/vac_programs.pdf.
   Courtesy of David Lalman, PhD, Department of Animal Science, Oklahoma State University, Stillwater, OK.

value-added management practices. Thus, the cow-calf industry has seen incomplete adoption of value-added management practices. Many concerns exist among cow-calf producers with regard to adoption of various value-added management practices. Many producers perceive that the price premiums accrue more often to larger producers. In addition, many producers seek to be low-cost producers and are hesitant to invest in potentially higher-cost rearing strategies. Williams and colleagues[24] used matching pairs to calculate differences in premiums and net returns between producers already using value-added management practices and those who do not (nonadopters). The goal of the investigators was to assess the likelihood that a producer would receive a premium for a set of value-added practices and to compute the likelihood of positive economic returns to the adoption of those practices. In short, the likelihood of positive premiums and net returns for individual practices and practice bundles are calculated. The average treatment effect for the producers who already adopted a practice was $4.93/cwt, $5.40/cwt, and $5.36/cwt for weaning, vaccinating, and dehorning, respectively. Also, the average treatment or price the nonadopters would have received if they performed the procedure was $5.80/cwt, $8.02/cwt, and $3.77/cwt for weaning, vaccinating, and dehorning, respectively. Bundles of attributes were evaluated, and the values were less than the sum of the individual premiums for the practices. The mean calculated average treatment effect for weaning was $5.13/cwt, and a producer was estimated to receive a positive premium 59% of the time. In addition to estimating the probability of a positive premium, costs were incorporated into the analysis to allow calculation of the probability of a positive net return. The probability of positive net returns ranges from 57% for dehorning to 79% for certified VAC45 program, and probabilities increase with more practices adopted. By taking into account the potential premiums and estimated cost, this analysis facilitates understanding of the likely economic impacts of adoption of value-added practices for cow-calf producers. Going beyond traditional analyses of this kind, this work also takes into account the variation in expected returns to estimate the likelihood of premiums and returns being realized by producers, which facilitates informed decision making with their study showing a positive net return for the procedures analyzed.

Advantages of Feeding Preconditioned Calves

Buyers are willing to pay more for calves if their likelihood of profitability increases. In fact, most studies show that PC calves generally sell below their full added value. Research by Cravey[25] with 380 PC calves compared with 1600 unweaned calves showed a net value difference of $60.72 or $11.04/cwt for the PC calves in the feedlot.[25] PC calves had less days on feed, higher ADG, and improved feed:gain with decreased morbidity, medicine cost, and mortality. In a second and similar experiment, Cravey (1996)[25] compared 15 lots of PC calves to 15 non-PC calves and similar advantages were identified for PC calves. In this study, the PC calves had a morbidity rate of 19%, whereas the non-PC calves had a morbidity rate of 62%. PC calves were worth $55.93 more/head or $9.67/cwt than non-PC calves because of factors listed in the previous study. In both cases, calves were sold on a live weight basis, so no additional value due to potential carcass quality premiums was included. This study showed that the full value of PC heifers was $9.67/cwt to $11.04/cwt when in that same year PC calves sold at a health sales price advantage of only $3.35/cwt.[22,25]

The primary reason that buyers are willing to pay a premium for PC calves is that they have a higher potential for profit in the feedlot, predominantly because of their decreased risk of morbidity and mortality due to bovine respiratory disease (BRD), which has been shown in many studies.[3,25–28]

Calves with improved health tend to have higher ADG, decreased cost of gain, and improved profitability compared with calves that become moribund.[3,25,27,28] Studies that include carcass data show an improvement in marbling, quality grade, and hot carcass weight in calves that remain healthy versus those treated one or more times for BRD.[3,27–29] Calves treated one or more times for BRD do tend to have lower yield grades primarily because of decreased fat thickness.[27,29] The effects of morbidity on performance, carcass quality, and profitability are clearly demonstrated in data collected on over 16,000 head of cattle in the Texas Ranch to Rail program (Table 4).[2]

Data from the Texas Ranch to Rail program show that the timing and type of vaccination affects feedlot morbidity and mortality. In their studies, calves that receive 2 doses of Modified live virus (MLV) BRD vaccine containing IBR-BVD-PI$_3$-BRSV with the initial dose given at least 9 weeks before weaning show the lowest morbidity and mortality when compared with those that receive alternative immunization protocols. If calves enter the feedlot with 2 doses of MLV BRD vaccine given at label

Table 4 Texas ranch to rail findings			
Item	Healthy	Sick	Difference
Number of cattle	12.306	4.047	—
Medicine/treatment cost	0	27.03	27.03
ADG (lb)[a]	2.99	2.67	0.32
Net return/head ($)[a]	67.32	−20.28	87.60
USDA choice or higher (%)[a]	39.6	27.5	11.1
USDA standard, (%)[b]	5.25	10.0	4.75

Calves were considered sick if they received one or more treatments for BRD.
Abbreviation: USDA, US Department of Agriculture.
[a] Healthy versus sick differs $P \le .01$.
[b] Healthy versus sick differs $P = .02$.
Courtesy of David Lalman, PhD, Department of Animal Science, Oklahoma State University, Stillwater, OK.

recommendation of at least 3 weeks between doses and the final dose at least 3 weeks before feedlot entry, there is little evidence to support any additional BRD immunizations.[30] This fact can save the feedlot owner money and labor when receiving and acclimating new cattle while decreasing stress for the cattle.

In work at the Tri-County Steer Carcass Futurity in Iowa, nonweaned calves were 3.4 times more likely to experience BRD than calves weaned greater than 30 days and calves given killed vaccine were 2.2 times more likely to get sick when compared with calves given MLV vaccine.[29]

Most PC protocols call for an initial dose of BRD vaccine to be given 3 to 4 weeks preweaning with a follow-up dose given the day of weaning. While the immunization at weaning creates little additional labor requirement, the preweaning injection often requires an additional processing time creating additional labor needs. On many beef farms and ranches, the lack of available labor is a common answer to questions about why calves are not PC. A study by Kirkpatrick and colleagues[31] demonstrated no differences in outcomes between vaccinating calves at approximately 2 months of age and again at weaning and vaccinating them at approximately 3 weeks before weaning and again at weaning in terms of immunologic response and treatment costs. Many times calves are already walking through the chute at approximately 2 months of age to be vaccinated (potentially with clostridial products), fly tagged, castrated if not done at birth, hot-iron dehorned if horned, and implanted with a growth stimulant. Giving the initial BRD vaccine at this time becomes a good management procedure to save time and labor without sacrificing outcomes.

The supply of PC calves continues to increase, and demand continues to outpace supply with PC premiums increasing each year.[22,23] The most obvious reason for this is that feedlot owners improve profitability due to enhanced health, growth, feed efficiency, and/or carcass quality of the calves. The true value of PC calves allows cow-calf producers to market PC calves at prices superior to non-PC calves.

Enhanced animal welfare
A factor that does not receive enough attention in the debate of purchasing PC versus high-risk cattle is the animal welfare aspect. The public is increasingly interested in how their food is raised. Using a best management practice such as PC can be easily championed when explaining the goal of decreased morbidity and mortality to the

over 98% of the US population not directly involved in agriculture. It is simply the right thing to do, and our livestock deserve to have the best care at all times in their life.

SUMMARY

There has been little disagreement that PC calves improves the subsequent health of these calves in the feedlot. Additional studies have shown benefits to ADG, feed efficiency, and carcass quality. The longstanding question has been if it is financially viable for the cow-calf producer to spend the time and money to produce the PC calf for the feedlot. Although the PC health sales price advantage has grown substantially over the past 20 years, focusing only on this premium gives an incomplete economic picture of the process. Factors that are under the control of the producer generally provide greater and more predictable economic return to the cow-calf owner. Weight gain of the calves, length of the PC period, and selection of marketing options are all factors that can greatly impact the profitability of producing PC calves.

REFERENCES

1. Patrick T. Launch First Iowa Program on pre-conditioning of cattle. Des Moines (IA): The Des Moines Register; 1967.
2. Lalman D, Mourer G. Effects of preconditioning on health, performance and prices of weaned calves. Oklahoma State University Cooperative Extension Service Bulletin F-3529. 2014. Available at: http://pods.dasnr.okstate.edu/docushare/dsweb/Get/Document-2013/ANSI-3529web.pdf.%202002. Accessed October 5, 2014.
3. Ensley DT. Attitudes and experiences with the Iowa Beef Cattle Preconditioning Program: a survey of feedlot operators [Master's thesis]. Ames (IA): Iowa State University Library; 2001.
4. Meyer KB, Judy JW Jr, Armstrong JH. Economic analysis of a feeder cattle preconditioning program. J Am Vet Med Assoc 1970;157:1560.
5. Cole NA. Preconditioning calves for the feedlot. Vet Clin North Am Food Anim Pract 1985;1:401.
6. Avent RK, Ward CE, Lalman DL. Market valuation of preconditioning feeder calves. J Agric Appl Econ 2004;36:173–83.
7. Boyles SL, Loerch SC, Lowe GD. Effects of weaning management strategies on performance and health of calves during feedlot receiving. Prof Anim Sci 2007; 23:637–41.
8. Dhuyvetter KC, Bryant AM, Blasi DA. Case study: preconditioning beef calves: are expected premiums sufficient to justify the practice? Prof Anim Sci 2005;21:502–14.
9. Dhuyvetter KC. Economics of preconditioning calves. Paper presented at the 2004 Kansas State University Agricultural Lenders Conference. Kansas State University. Manhattan (KS), October 29, 2004.
10. Mathis CP, Cox SH, Löest CA, et al. Pasture preconditioning calves at a higher rate of gain improves feedlot health but not postweaning profit. Prof Anim Sci 2009;25:475–80.
11. Barnes K, Smith S, Lalman DL. Managing shrink and weighing conditions in beef cattle. Oklahoma Coop. Ext. Serv. ANSI-3257. 2007. Available at: http://osufacts.okstate.edu. Accessed November 27, 2014.
12. Pritchard RH, Mendez JK. Effects of preconditioning on pre-and post-shipment performance of feeder calves. J Anim Sci 1990;68(1):28–34.
13. Bailey D, Stenquist NJ. Preconditioning calves for feedlots. Managing for Today's Cattle Market and Beyond. Tuscon (AZ): Livestock Marketing Information Center

(LMIC); 1996. Available at: http://ag.arizona.edu/arec/wemc/TodaysCattlePub. html. Accessed October 6, 2014.

14. Hilton WM, Olynk NJ. Profitability of preconditioning: lessons learned from an eleven-year study of an Indiana beef herd. Bov Pract 2011;45:40–50.

15. Rawls E. Can you afford to wean and feed your calves? Tennessee Beef Cattle Initiative. 2002. Available at: http://www.tnbeefcattleinitiative.org/production.htm. Accessed November 17, 2014.

16. Donnell JD. Age and source verified preconditioned feeder cattle: costs and value [Master's thesis]. Stillwater (OK): Oklahoma State University; 2007.

17. Historic Cash Corn Prices. Available at: http://www.extension.iastate.edu/agdm/ crops/pdf/a2-11.pdf. Accessed December 26, 2014.

18. Historic Alfalfa Hay Prices. Available at: http://future.aae.wisc.edu/data/monthly_ values/by_area/2053?area=US. Accessed December 26, 2014.

19. Historic Cattle Prices - Iowa State University Extension and Outreach. Available at: http://www.extension.iastate.edu/agdm/livestock/pdf/b2-12.pdf. Accessed December 26, 2014.

20. Schulz L, Dhuyvetter K, Harborth K, et al. Factors affecting feeder cattle prices in Kansas and Missouri. Cooperative Extension Service. Manhattan (KS): Kansas State University; 2010. Available at: www.agmangerinfo.net. Accessed November 17, 2014.

21. Barham BL, Troxel TR. Factors affecting the selling price of feeder cattle sold at Arkansas livestock auctions in 2005. J Anim Sci 2007;85:3434–41.

22. King ME, Salman MD, Wittum TE, et al. Effect of certified health programs on the sale price of beef calves marketed through a livestock videotape auction service from 1995 through 2005. J Am Vet Med Assoc 2006;229:1389–400.

23. Seeger JT, King ME, Grotelueschen DM, et al. Effect of management, marketing, and certified health programs on the sale price of beef calves sold through a live-stock video auction service from 1995 through 2009. J Am Vet Med Assoc 2011; 239(4):451–66.

24. Williams BR, DeVuyst EA, Peel DS, et al. The likelihood of positive returns from value-added calf management practices. J Agric Appl Econ 2014;46:125–38.

25. Cravey M. Preconditioning effect on feedlot performance. Proc Southwest Nutr Management Conf. Phoenix, AZ. 1996. p. 33–7.

26. Roeber DL, Speer NC, Gentry JG, et al. Feeder cattle health management: effects on morbidity rates, feedlot performance, carcass characteristics, and beef palatability. The Professional Animal Scientist 2001;17(1):39–44.

27. Schneider MJ, Tait RG Jr, Busby WD, et al. An evaluation of bovine respiratory disease complex in feedlot cattle: impact on performance and carcass traits using treatment records and lung lesion scores. J Anim Sci 2009;87:1821–7.

28. Gardner BA, Dolezal HG, Owens FN, et al. Impact of health on profitability of feedlot steers. Okla Agr Exp Sta Res Rep 1998;P-965:102.

29. Busby D. Tri-county steer futurity data. Proc Am Assoc Bov Pract Conf. 2010. p. 71–81.

30. Lalman D, Smith R. Effects of preconditioning on health, performance and prices of weaned calves. Oklahoma State University Cooperative Extension Service Bulletin F-3529. 2002. Available at: http://pods.dasnr.okstate.edu/docushare/ dsweb/Get/Document-2013/ANSI-3529web.pdf. Accessed June 10, 2010.

31. Kirkpatrick JG, Step DL, Payton ME, et al. Effect of age at the time of vaccination on antibody titers and feedlot performance in beef calves. J Am Vet Med Assoc 2008;233(1):136–42.

Management of Pregnant Heifers in the Feedlot

Ryan D. Rademacher, DVM, Brian N. Warr, DVM, Calvin W. Booker, DVM, MVetSc*

KEYWORDS

- Pregnant heifer • Feedlot • Abortifacients

KEY POINTS

- Managing pregnant heifers in the feedlot poses many economic and animal health/welfare challenges for feedlot producers.
- The mainstay of many pregnant heifer management strategies is the use of abortifacients early in the feeding period.
- In instances where pregnancy diagnosis of individual animals is not practical, group-level management strategies may be implemented.
- Feedlot operators should be aware of the economic liabilities associated with feeding pregnant heifers so that they can make informed purchase and management decisions.

INTRODUCTION

Pregnancy in the feedlot heifer presents several undesirable issues to the cattle owner and feedlot operator. An obvious disadvantage is the associated calving complications when heifers reach parturition while on feed (including dystocia, retained fetal membranes, peripheral nerve paralysis, and mortality).[1,2] In addition, heifers that are pregnant at slaughter tend to have decreased average daily gain (ADG) when adjusting for pregnancy weight,[3] inferior feed/gain ratio (F:G) on a carcass-adjusted basis,[3,4] decreased dressing percent,[3–8] and lower slaughter values[1,6] as compared with heifers not pregnant at the time of slaughter. **Table 1** summarizes studies that have evaluated the effect of pregnancy status on feedlot performance.

On a live-weight basis, heifers pregnant at slaughter have been demonstrated to have improved[7] or equivalent[8] ADG as compared with heifers that were open. Additionally, on a live-weight basis, heifers pregnant at arrival to the feedlot and not aborted had improved feed to gain as compared with heifers open on arrival[3] and pregnant heifers aborted at arrival.[3,4] This finding is largely attributed to the increase in fetal, uterine, and fluid weight associated with pregnancy.[3,5] However,

The authors have nothing to disclose.
Feedlot Health Management Services Ltd, PO Box 140, Okotoks, Alberta T1S 2A2, Canada
* Corresponding author.
E-mail address: calvinb@feedlothealth.com

Table 1
Summary of studies evaluating performance of pregnant heifers

Study	Population	ADG[a]	F:G[b]	HCW	Dressing Percent
Bishop et al,[8] 2003	Open: fed 105 or 147 d (n = 43)	—	—	799 lb	62.6%[c]
	Pregnant: 60 d gestation, fed 105 or 147 d (n = 25)	—	—	777 lb	60.3%[d]
Kreikemeier et al,[9] 1993	Open at slaughter (n = 6565)	—	—	296 kg[c]	—
	Second trimester at slaughter (n = 208)	—	—	291 kg[d]	—
	Third trimester at slaughter (n = 185)	—	—	292 kg[d]	—
Jim et al,[3] 1991[f]	Open: fed 91 d (n = 48)	1.62 kg[c] SD ± 0.07	7.45[c] SD ± 0.08	310.6 kg[c]	55.43%[c] SD ± 0.51
	Aborted: 91–144 d gestation, fed 91 d (n = 47)	1.47 kg[d] SD ± 0.06	7.92[c] SD ± 0.26	300.9 kg[d]	55.03%[c] SD ± 0.57
	Pregnant: 91–144 d gestation, fed 91 d (n = 48)	1.26 kg[e] SD ± 0.09	9.37[d] SD ± 0.65	289.8 kg[e]	51.73%[d] SD ± 0.70
Stanton et al,[4] 1988[g]	Aborted: 145 d gestation, fed 91 d (n = 30)	2.63 lb	8.38[c]	—	59.72%[c]
	Pregnant: 145 d gestation, fed 91 d (n = 30)	2.42 lb	9.46[d]	—	54.48%[d]
Bennett et al,[5] 1984[h]	Lots with 0% pregnant at slaughter (n = 5004)	—	—	—	63.3%
	Lots with mean 23.3% pregnant at slaughter (n = 5016)	—	—	—	62.0%
Edwards & Laudert,[7] 1984	Aborted: fed 105 d (n = 115)	—	—	566 lb[c]	61.6%[c]
	Pregnant at slaughter: fed 105 d (n = 39)	—	—	546 lb[d]	57.6%[d]

Abbreviation: HCW, hot carcass weight.
[a] ADG presented in either pounds per day or kilograms per day based on study.
[b] F:G is the amount of feed on a dry-matter basis required in pounds or kgs to generate 1 pound or 1 kg of gain, respectively.
[c,d,e] Values from same study lacking a common superscript are significantly different (P<.05).
[f] Values for ADG and F:G based on adjusted live weight (live weight minus uterine weight at slaughter).
[g] Values for ADG and F:G based on carcass-adjusted weights (assuming 50% dress on initial weight).
[h] No statistical analysis reported.

carcass-adjusted ADG in pregnant heifers has been shown to be lower than that of aborted and open heifers.[3,4] Jim and colleagues[3] also reported that adjusted live-weight-basis ADG was lower in aborted heifers than heifers that were not pregnant at arrival to the feedlot.

Carcass-adjusted F:G in heifers pregnant at slaughter is worse than that of heifers not pregnant at the time of slaughter (either aborted or open at arrival to the feedlot).[3,4]

This increase in pregnancy-associated weight also shows up as decreased dressing percent and lower hot carcass weights for heifers pregnant at slaughter[3,7,9] and those that have recently calved.[7] Intuitively, as the stage of gestation increases, the dressing percent decreases further.[5,7] One study that characterized the total weight attributed to the gravid uterus by stage in gestation showed that a 210-day pregnancy at slaughter equaled 56 lb (25.4 kg) (**Table 2**).[5] In another study, the mean total uterine weight at slaughter was 34.0 kg (SD = 8.9; range 14.1–57.2 kg) and the mean fetal age was 225 days (SD = 16; range 175–252).[3] Even when heifers are marketed live, the obvious presence of pregnant heifers or a history of delivering considerable numbers of pregnant heifers may result in lower bids/sale prices.[1,6]

The prevalence of pregnancy in heifers entering the feedlot is variable and depends on a variety of factors such as season, cattle source, and industry trends. Data reported by Edwards and Laudert[7] from 20,526 and 19,924 heifers entering a single feedlot in 1982 and 1983, respectively, revealed that pregnancy rates tended to be higher in the late winter and early spring. A second study in which random lots of heifers originating from Kansas feedlots and slaughtered at 5 different packing plants in Kansas during 1986 to 1987 (82,733 animal) revealed that the highest prevalence of pregnant heifers at slaughter occurred during the months of November to March.[10] A summary of studies evaluating pregnancy prevalence in feedlot heifers at arrival and at slaughter is summarized in **Table 3**. For practical purposes, retrospective data for each individual production system may serve as a valuable indicator of pregnancy risk among incoming groups of heifers.

MANAGEMENT OPTIONS

Feedlot arrival protocols should be previously validated as to achieve a predictable and uniform outcome across the entire pen or lot. These strategies must also consider animal welfare and cost-effectiveness before implementation. A large variety of management options for pregnant heifers exist (**Box 1**). Only those presented in previous studies or commonly used by industry are included in this review. On an individual feedlot basis, there may be other options that are better suited to meet the needs of specific operations; however, these go beyond the scope of this review. Although there are some situations in which nothing is done to manage pregnant heifers entering the feedlot, the mainstay of many management strategies is the use abortifacients to terminate pregnancies early in the feeding period.[11] Selection of abortifacients should be determined by the stage of pregnancy and is discussed in more detail in a later section of this article.

When determining the most appropriate protocol for incoming heifers, it is important to factor the relative economics of different management decisions for the individual group of heifers. Multiple studies have estimated the economic liability associated with feeding pregnant heifers (**Table 4**). Although providing an economic model for the decision process, these analyses must be viewed cautiously as multiple factors

Table 2							
Weight loss attributed to pregnancy at slaughter							
Days Gestation	90	120	150	180	210	240	Term
Weight loss (lb)	1	9	17	30	56	106	180

Data from Bennett BW, Clayton RP, Cravens RL, et al. Slaughter weight loss attributable to pregnancy in feedlot heifers. Mod Vet Pract 1984;65:677–9.

Table 3
Summary of studies evaluating prevalence of pregnancies in heifers at arrival to the feedlot or at time of slaughter

Study	Year	Population	Pregnancy Prevalence (%)
Pregnancy Prevalence on Arrival to Feedlot			
USDA, 2012[11]	2011	Randomized survey of feedlots with greater than 1000 head capacity in 12 US states	7.6
Data presented in Laudert, 1988	1987	58,000 Heifers at one feedlot	4.4
	1986	40,000 Heifers at one feedlot	6.0
Data presented in Bennett, 1985	1983	Survey of Colorado feeders	16.5
Data presented in Edwards & Laudert,[7]	1983	19,924 Heifers at one feedlot	9.0
1984	1982	20,526 Heifers at one feedlot	15.0
Pregnancy Prevalence at Slaughter			
Kreikemeier et al,[9] 1993	1990 (January–April)	8292 Heifers from 23 yards (northern Texas, western Oklahoma & Kansas, eastern Colorado & New Mexico) at a packing plant in southwest Kansas	4.74 (Range: 0–25)
Laudert,[10] 1988	1986–1987	82,733 Heifers from Kansas yards at 5 Kansas packing plants	3.93
	1986–1987	24,658 Heifers from Colorado yards at 5 Kansas packing plants	4.1
Bennett et al,[5] 1984	November 1983, late January–February 1984	Lots containing pregnant heifers (5016 heifers) Monfort Packing Plant, Greely, CO (does not include lots with no pregnant heifers during same time period)	23.3
	November 1983, late January–February 1984	Lots containing pregnant heiferettes (507 heiferettes) Monfort Packing Plant, Greely, CO (does not include lots with no pregnant heifers during same time period)	22.9
Data presented in Bennett,[12] 1985	1983	Survey of Colorado packing plants	17

Abbreviation: USDA, US Department of Agriculture.

Box 1
Summary of common options to manage pregnant heifers

- Do not feed heifers[1]
- Purchase guaranteed open or spayed heifers[1,7,12]
- Purchase heifers, introduce no management strategy for pregnant heifers, and deal with problems as they arise[12,13]
- Observe heifer pens, and ship or sort off obviously pregnant heifers before calving[1,7]
- Administer an abortifacient to all heifers at or soon after arrival[1,13]
- Diagnose pregnancy at or soon after arrival
  - Administer abortifacients to animals determined to be pregnant at or soon after arrival[1,12,13]
  - Return or sell heifers determined to be pregnant[12]
  - Retain pregnant heifers in feedlot but market before expected parturition (authors' observations)
  - Calve out pregnant heifers separately (authors' observations)

---

affect the economics of feeding pregnant heifers. Pregnancy rate within the lot or group is one of the most important factors driving this decision. In a simulation model developed by Buhman and colleagues,[13] administering abortifacients to all heifers regardless of pregnancy status was more economical at high pregnancy rates ($\geq$43%) compared with palpating and aborting only those pregnant.[13] However, when pregnancy rates were 36% or less, palpating and aborting became the most economical option.[13] It is not until pregnancy rates approach 0% that doing nothing to manage pregnant heifers becomes the most economical option.[13]

Pregnant heifers introduce additional cost to the system. Regardless of the strategy implemented, it is important to understand that when purchase price for the same weight heifers is equivalent, aborting heifers will result in lower returns than feeding heifers that were never pregnant to start with.[3,12,13] Performance expectations from available research must be considered along with current economic/market conditions in order to determine the most cost-effective strategy for each situation.

PREGNANCY DIAGNOSIS

In order to determine if pregnancy diagnosis and abortion of only pregnant animals is a cost-effective management decision, the available pregnancy diagnosis options must be considered. Options that may be available to a producer include transrectal palpation, transrectal ultrasonography, and serum pregnancy tests. Each of these methods has advantages as well as limitations that should be considered in full. Accuracy of transrectal ultrasonography (Thomas Edwards, DVM, Kearney, NE, personal communication, 2014) and palpation may be impacted by skill and experience of the examiner, age of the heifer, size of the heifer, and other factors (authors' observations).[14]

An incorrect pregnancy diagnosis (false positives and false negatives) will result in economic loss to the feedlot. The cost of a false positive will be determined by how animals diagnosed as pregnant are managed. This cost may include, but is not limited to, the cost of marketing if pregnant heifers are to be sold or cost of unnecessary abortifacient administration. Conversely, the cost of a false negative will be determined by the cost of production losses, including calving complications, associated with

Table 4
Summary of studies evaluating the economics of different management strategies for pregnant heifers

Study Description	Assumptions	Results

Buhman et al,[13] 2003
 	
Simulation using a partial budget and dynamic model to evaluate 3 management decisions: palpate and abort, abort all, nothing
	• Purchase weight of 318 kg
	• 200 Animal pens with a mean 10% pregnant
	• Mean 50% of heifers that remained pregnant calve in the feedlot
	• $2 Palpation cost per heifer palpated
	• $3.50 Abortifacient cost per heifer aborted
	• 95% Efficacy of abortifacients
	• Mean 5% increase in BRD morbidity risk for aborted heifers (above normal morbidity)
	• 2% Abortion-related health risk; $3 per sick heifer
	• 15% Dystocia (percent of pregnant); $13 per treatment
	• 3% Caesarian section (percent of pregnant); $85 per procedure
	• 6% Pregnancy-related death (percent of pregnant)
	• Fed for 160 DOF
	• Feed cost $114.57/ton DM
	• Sell baby calves from 50% of calvers; $100 per calf
	• Open heifer pay weight: 544 kg (63.5% dress)
	• Pregnant heifer pay weight: 544 kg (59.8% dress)
	• Recently calved heifers pay weight: 454 kg (63.5% dress)
	• Open heifer price drawn from distributions derived from annual mean prices in 20-y historical database
	• $10.00 Lower rail price for pregnant heifers; all other heifer prices the same
		5th–95th percentile net returns
		Open heifers
		  Marketed live
		    • −$58.14 to $170.57
		  Marketed on rail
		    • −$45.01 to $192.50
		Pregnant heifers
		  Marketed live
		    • −$162.32 to $43.57
		  Marketed on rail
		    • −$267.57 to −$66.60
		Aborted heifers
		  Marketed live
		    • −$69.75 to $152.02
		  Marketed on rail
		    • −$63.70 to $171.16
		The bid price for finished cattle and DOF had largest effect on net return. Pregnancy-related death loss was also important for pregnant heifers.

Jim et al,[3] 1991
 	
Economic analysis based on field trial results
	• HCW: open = 310.6 kg, aborted = 300.9 kg, and pregnant heifers = 289.8 kg; $3.19/kg HCW
	• $6.00 Per animal aborting cost
	• $2.00 Per animal palpation cost
	• $1.00 Per animal labor cost
	• Costs associated with managing complications of induced abortion (labor, morbidity, mortality, and so forth) were assumed to be equivalent to the costs associated with managing calving complications in pregnant heifers
		Aborted heifers
		  Returned $26.41 per animal more than pregnant heifers
		Open heifers
		  Returned $39.94 per animal and $66.35 per animal more than aborted and pregnant heifers, respectively

Study	Details	Outcomes
Stanton et al,[4] 1988 *Economic analysis based on field trial results*	• Pregnant heifers had a 1.03 lb/d increase in DM feed intake over a 91-d feeding period (feed cost: $0.07/lb DM) compared with aborted heifers • Pregnant heifers had a 15.5 lb lighter carcass (sale price of $0.92/lb HCW) compared with aborted heifers • Cost for aborting included: late-term abortifacients ($4.00 per animal), palpation ($2.00 per animal), and treatment of retained placentas ($4.46 per animal prorated across aborted heifers) • Does not account for many factors, such as mortality differences, calving complications, and abortion complications	A net economic advantage of $10.36 per animal existed for aborting late-term heifers

Bennett,[12] 1985
Economic modeling based on retrospective slaughter data and previous research
	• 1000 Animals per decision
	• 16.5% Pregnancy rate on arrival
	• Taken to a 1000-lb slaughter weight
	• Heifers open or pregnant at slaughter achieved a dressing percent of 63.3% or 60.3%, respectively
	• Sale price of $100.00/cwt HCW
	• All heifers that calved or needed abortion treatment were hospitalized for 3 d at cost of $5.00/d
	• Calving loss per animal of $157.47
	• Dead animal loss reported to be $58.00/cwt
	• Palpation charge of $2.00 per animal
	• Feed cost of $140.00/ton
	3 Simulated management choices
	• Do nothing
	   Pregnant heifers: 8% decrease in ADG, 110 lb of additional feed, 41 of 165 calve during the feeding period with 10 that die of calving complications
	• Palpate and abort
	   Increased labor cost of $0.16 per animal, 80% efficacy of abortifacients, $3.29 per animal abortifacient cost, 10% of aborting heifers need treatment
	   Aborted heifers: 4% decreased ADG, 99 lb of additional feed in aborted heifers, 8 heifers calve during the feeding period, 2 of the 8 heifers that calve would die of calving complications
	• Palpate and sell back
	   $2.00 per animal palpation cost, sell back price = purchase price minus $4.00/cwt, estimated yardage + insurance + commission + and so forth = $2000
		Do nothing
		$115.42 loss per pregnant heifer ($19.04 loss per heifer)
		Palpate and abort
		$52.76 loss per pregnant heifer ($8.71 loss per heifer)
		Palpate and sell back
		$50.24 loss per pregnant heifer ($8.29 loss per heifer)

(continued on next page)

Table 4
(continued)

Study Description	Assumptions	Results
Edwards & Laudert,[7] 1984 *Economic analysis based on field trial results*	• A 100% pregnancy rate was used for all groups • 4% Of aborted heifers pregnant at slaughter • 44% Of nonaborted heifers pregnant at slaughter • 8% Of nonaborted heifers had recently calved at time of slaughter • Aborted heifers: HCW = 615 lb (61.4% dress) • Pregnant heifers: HCW = 598 lb (59.6% dress) • Sale price of $100.00/cwt HCW • Does not account for palpation/abortion costs, labor costs, mortality differences, or performance differences	A $17.00 per animal gross economic benefit for aborted heifers vs non aborted heifers when solely accounting for gain and dressing percentage

Abbreviations: BRD, bovine respiratory disease; cwt, hundred weight; DM, dry matter; DOF, days on feed; dress, dressing percent.

feeding a pregnant animal. No method of pregnancy diagnosis is accurate in very early gestation (generally <30 days depending on the method of pregnancy determination). Therefore, one must consider the following scenario: If a heifer that arrives to the feedlot at 30 days' gestation is misdiagnosed as open and fed for 150 days, a 180-day pregnancy at slaughter can be expected to result in 30 lb of pregnancy-associated weight,[5] which will be reflected as a decreased dressing percent and poorer F:G on a carcass-adjusted basis. As a result, one management option may be to delay the pregnancy diagnosis until the minimum days on feed that allows for accurate diagnosis of the entire group of heifers[1] realizing that aborting heifers later in gestation may result in more complications[2] and increased performance cost.[1,4]

A final consideration of cost associated with a pregnancy diagnosis is the possibility of decreased throughput at the processing facility and inefficiencies associated with trying to synchronize the examiner or sample collector with the processing crew's schedule (authors' observations). The following are practical options for pregnancy diagnosis in the feedlot.

Transrectal Palpation

A major advantage of transrectal palpation for pregnancy diagnosis is that it provides a real-time assessment so that management can be executed at the time of processing. It is generally accepted that palpation per rectum can be used to accurately diagnose pregnancies from as early as 30 days after conception through the rest of gestation.[14] In dairy cows, Warnick and colleagues[15] demonstrated that approximately 4.8% of cows diagnosed as open at the first pregnancy examination (≥30 days after breeding) by veterinarians in 32 New York dairy herds were actually pregnant at the time of rectal palpation based on subsequent calving date.[15] Approximately 3.4% of cows diagnosed as pregnant at the first pregnancy examination (≥30 days after breeding) were later rebred; 1.5% diagnosed as pregnant at the first pregnancy diagnosis were later diagnosed as open at the time of reexamination. (The authors acknowledge that dairy cows are different than beef heifers; however, this citation provides quantitative measurement of rectal palpation accuracy.)[15] The cost associated with palpation may be highly variable, as some production systems may rely on a veterinarian for palpation and will pay for professional services. Other systems may have the option of using a trained member of the feedlot crew. However, it is necessary to make sure that this option does not conflict with local veterinary practice laws.

Transrectal Ultrasonography

Similar to transrectal palpation, transrectal ultrasonography provides a real-time diagnosis of pregnancy. Linear-array transducers of both 5-MHz and 7-MHz frequency ranges are commonly used for transrectal ultrasonography,[14,16] and a 5-MHZ transducer is generally accepted as being an accurate method for diagnosing pregnancy after day 24.[14] Ultrasonography has the potential to identify positive signs of pregnancy earlier than transrectal palpation. Pierson and Ginther[17] have described identification of the embryonic vesicle in Holstein heifers between days 12 and 14 using a 5-MHz probe. However, ultrasonography accuracy is noted to increase with days of gestation.[16,18,19]

With decreasing technology cost, ultrasonography may be economically practical in certain production systems; professional fees for ultrasound pregnancy diagnosis are generally comparable with the fees for transrectal palpation (authors' observations). The cost of purchasing portable ultrasound equipment suitable for a feedlot operation ranges from $6500 to $13,500 (Thomas Edwards, DVM, Kearney, NE, personal communication, 2014). The per-animal pregnancy diagnosis cost is variable and depends on the true depreciation and labor costs associated with operating the machine at each operation. With the addition of an introducer arm, the operator is no longer required to manually enter the rectum, which has the potential to reduce injuries to cattle and examiner while potentially increasing the speed of diagnosis (Thomas Edwards, DVM, Kearney, NE, personal communication, 2014).[20]

Biochemical Pregnancy Tests

Multiple biochemical tests have been described, including serum progesterone, estrone sulfate, bovine pregnancy-specific protein B (bPSPB), and immunosuppressive early pregnancy factor.[14] Of these, bPSPB is currently the only commercially available test that may have application in feedlot heifer management. bPSPB is released by trophoblastic cells in cows and can be detected as early as 15 days after insemination and in nearly all pregnant cows by 24 days after insemination.[14] The concentration of bPSPB increases as days of gestation increase and is present until parturition. Examples of current commercially available tests include BioPRYN and BioPRYN QK offered by BioTracking Laboratory (Moscow, ID), IDEXX Bovine Pregnancy Test and IDEXX Visual Pregnancy test offered by IDEXX (Westbrook ME), and the DG29 Bovine Pregnancy Test offered by Conception Animal Reproduction Technologies (Beaumont, QC, Canada).[20,21] Each test has similar requirements and, in general, require that the animals be at least 28 to 29 days of gestation for accurate results.[20,21] The BioPRYN test claims to have a 1% false-negative rate and a 5% false-positive rate,[22] whereas IDEXX claims 99.3% sensitivity and 95.1% specificity.[23] A major consideration in using a serum test to diagnosis pregnancy in feedlot heifers is that the pregnancy status will not be determined at the time of sample collection. As a result, management considerations have to be made in order to determine when to abort animals diagnosed as pregnant. The listed options have various lag times in test results, the shortest being IDEXX Visual Pregnancy test, which takes 2 hours from set up.[23] The cost varies by test but ranges from $2.50 to $3.50 per sample.[21,22]

PHARMACOLOGIC ABORTIFACIENT STRATEGIES

The efficacies of the different pharmacologic abortifacient strategies have been well documented to vary based on stage of gestation. As a result, the pharmacologic approach to termination of pregnancy using a single abortifacient depends on the stage of gestation.[1,7,24–26] When dexamethasone and prostaglandins are used in combination they have been determined to be effective at all stages of pregnancy.[27] Abortifacient strategy may be determined on the individual animal level based on one of the previously discussed pregnancy diagnosis options or at a group level. To understand the pharmacologic decision, it is important to review the physiologic processes involved in pregnancy maintenance. McDonald and colleagues[28] determined that maintenance of pregnancy in the bovine depends on the production of progesterone by the corpus luteum until at least day 150 of gestation. It was later summarized from multiple studies that bovine progesterone is luteal in origin until approximately 150 days of gestation and that the placenta acts as an additional progesterone source from day 150 to 250 days of gestation.[29] After day 250, the corpus luteum again assumes a primary role in the production of P4 for pregnancy maintenance.[29–31]

Commercial prostaglandin products are available and consist of dinoprost tromethamine, a naturally occurring prostaglandin marketed as Lutalyse,[32,33] and cloprostenol sodium, a prostaglandin analogue. Cloprostenol sodium is available in the United States and Canada as many commercially available products, which presently include estroPLAN,[34,38] Estrumate,[35,36] Juramate,[37] and Cloprostenol Veyx.[39] For discussion purposes, naturally occurring prostaglandin and prostaglandin analogue products are referred to collectively as a prostaglandin or prostaglandins in this summary. Prostaglandins administered at an appropriate dose have been demonstrated to reliably result in abortions in animals less than 150 days of gestation.[24,25,40] Day[25] further demonstrated that administration of the prostaglandin analogue cloprostenol sodium markedly reduced progesterone concentrations in all stages of gestation. Consistent with other studies, administration of 500 μg cloprostenol sodium resulted in abortion in 89.58% of cows that were less than 150 days' gestation, whereas cows beyond 150 days of gestation did not consistently abort.[25] These findings are supported by the normal physiology of pregnancy maintenance in the bovine; cloprostenol sodium regresses the corpus luteum structure; therefore, pregnancies less than 150 days of age are aborted. In feedlot heifers, it is generally considered that prostaglandins alone maintain appropriate efficacy until approximately day 150 of gestation, after which point, the sole use of these products is insufficient to consistently induce abortion.

Short-acting glucocorticoids, such as dexamethasone, have been demonstrated to mimic the increase of fetal cortisol[41,42] and, therefore, result in induced parturition for pregnancies greater than 225 days.[41–43] Dexamethasone may also act by suppressing the adrenal production of progesterone,[46] which has been presented as a nonluteal source of progesterone involved in bovine pregnancy maintenance.[31] Lauderdale[44] administered dexamethasone at a dosage of 20 mg/d for 3 days to Hereford, Aberdeen Angus, and Holstein cows at 185, 215, and 245 days of gestation and reported unsatisfactory abortion rates. Conversely, administration of prostaglandins to cows greater than 225 days of gestation has also been noted to reliably terminate pregnancies.[45] Similarly, the administration of prostaglandins on day 267 of gestation effectively shortened the gestation length in heifers.[40] As a result, pregnancies between 150 days and 255 days have an unpredictable response to the sole administration of either glucocorticoids or prostaglandins.

Termination of pregnancies later than 150 days' gestation is generally achieved through a combination therapy including both prostaglandins and dexamethasone. Johnson and colleagues[46] demonstrated that administration of 25 mg of dexamethasone and removal of the ovarian source of progesterone in cows that were 150 and 255 days' gestation produced a reliable method for pregnancy termination. Ovariectomy or administration of 500 μg cloprostenol sodium both proved to be adequate methods of removing the ovarian source of progesterone.[46]

In situations when the stage of gestation in pregnant heifers is accurately diagnosed, the feedlot has the option of administering the most appropriate drugs for the stage of pregnancy. When 23 feedlot veterinarians were surveyed, 78.26% responded that they recommended newly arrived heifers be examined for pregnancy status in some instances, emphasizing that those of unknown origin or management history be checked.[47] In many production systems, the cutoff for the maximum stage of gestation to administer only a prostaglandin for pregnancy termination is 120 days, therefore, allowing for a variation in diagnosis accuracy without sacrificing prostaglandin efficacy (authors' observation). In the previously mentioned survey, 34.87% of respondents recommended mass abortions without pregnancy checking for certain groups of heifers; most indicated appropriate candidates to be mixed-sex lots or heifers that arrived at the feedlot from August through December.[47] In situations when mass abortifacient administration occurs without pregnancy diagnosis, animal age or season of the year may be used to determine if the combination of dexamethasone and prostaglandin is warranted (authors' observations).

CLINICAL OUTCOMES

When used appropriately, abortifacient protocols are considered to provide good efficacy. Label claims for products containing cloprostenol sodium indicate that abortion rates of approximately 95% can be expected up to 4.5 months[35,37–39] to 5.0 months[34,36] of gestation. A similar label claim exists for dinoprost tromethamine in Canada.[32] However, in the United States, data from dinoprost tromethamine dose titration studies carried out at multiple sites were used to calculate a statistical predicted relative abortion rate of approximately 93% for the 5 mL (25 mg) dose up to 100 days of gestation.[33] Edwards and Laudert[7] showed that pregnant heifers administered the labeled doses of either cloprostenol sodium or dinoprost tromethamine before 120 days' gestation achieved abortion rates by day 20 after treatment of 93% and 85%, respectively.[7] Similar findings have been demonstrated by other studies.[3,24,43,48]

After day 150 of gestation, efficacy decreases when using a prostaglandin alone; therefore, dexamethasone should be used in conjunction with a prostaglandin.[1,7] In the previously mentioned study by Edwards and Laudert,[7] heifers greater than 120 days of gestation received either cloprostenol sodium (manufacturers' recommended dosage) + dexamethasone (20 mg) or dinoprost tromethamine (manufacturers' recommended dosage) + dexamethasone (20 mg); abortion rates on day 20 after treatment were 100% and 93% respectively. It is important to note that in this study, 14% of nontreated pregnant heifer controls had aborted by day 20 after treatment and only 44% remained pregnant at slaughter (7 of 85 controls had recently calved before slaughter).[7] In another study, the use of cloprostenol sodium (375 µg) + dexamethasone (20 mg) to abort heifers ranging from 91 to 144 days' gestation was 100% effective.[3] Barth and colleagues[27] reported success rates using a combination of cloprostenol sodium (500 µg) + dexamethasone (25 mg) at 1 to 4 months, 4 to 6 months, and 6 to 8 months of gestation to be 100%, 92.5%, and 92.5%, respectively. In this study, 2 of the failures in both the 4 to 6 month and 6 to 8 month groups were caused by fetal mummification. In another study, cloprostenol sodium (500 µg) + dexamethasone (20 mg) achieved abortion in 98% of the pregnant heifers by 5 days after induction (790 feedlot heifers of various gestation lengths, most being of first and second trimester).[2]

COMPLICATIONS AND CONCERNS

The practice of inducing abortion in pregnant feedlot heifers does not come without its own set of complications. Among these are failed abortions, retained placentas, metritis, potential for immunosuppression, human health concerns, and negative public perception. When using appropriate abortifacient protocols, failure to induce abortion will likely occur approximately 5.0% to 7.5% of the time as previously discussed.

Melengestrol acetate (MGA)[49,50] is commonly fed to feedlot heifers in order to suppress estrus behavior, and improve feedlot performance.[51–55] The labeled dosage of MGA for the suppression of estrus in feedlot heifers is 0.4 mg per animal per day in Canada[49] and 0.25 mg to 0.50 mg per animal per day in the United States,[50] with current recommended dosages in the range of 0.4 to 0.5 mg per animal per day.[51,53,54] Feeding of MGA during the period following administration of abortifacients has been implicated in reducing the success of induced abortion.[4] Studies evaluating the effect of feeding MGA on the efficacy of abortifacients are lacking, and information must be extrapolated from other investigations. In one study evaluating ovariectomized heifers, 9 of 13 heifers receiving 1.0 mg MGA daily remained pregnant after 30 days, whereas all 11 heifers that received a dosage of 0.4 mg/d or less had aborted by day 30.[56] Other studies have shown that daily injections of progesterone products following ovariectomy or corpus luteum ablation were successful in maintaining pregnancy.[28,57] Given the lack of direct evidence that MGA can be fed during the abortion period without consequence and inferences made from other studies on progesterone and pregnancy maintenance, it is considered a good management strategy to not begin feeding MGA until after heifers have aborted. Commonly, MGA is not included in the starter and step-up diets allowing adequate time for abortion to occur in a manner that is practical to implement at the feedlot level (authors' observations).

Heifers subjected to induced abortion protocols have higher frequency of complications, such as retained placentas (RP)[4,24,27] and fetal mummies.[27] Increased incidence of RP has also been observed with pharmaceutical induction of parturition in near-term pregnancies in primiparous heifers[43,58] and multiparous cows.[41,48,58] Comparisons between studies in the published literature is problematic because of the lack of a common definition for RP among studies. In one study evaluating different doses of cloprostenol sodium, 11 of 162 aborted heifers had RP as observed on day 9 after treatment.[24] When cloprostenol sodium and dexamethasone were used in combination, an 88% incidence of RP (retained >24 hours after expulsion of fetus) was observed.[27] The reported impact of RP is variable; however, the impact of uncomplicated RP is generally considered to be minimal. In 30 aborted heifers with a 43.3% incidence of RP, the average treatment cost at the time of this study (1991) was $10.31 per RP case.[4] However, other investigators report that the number of RP cases requiring treatment is low. No heifers required treatment in the previously mentioned study with 88% RP.[27] Although the incidence of RP is not presented, only 2 of 47 aborted heifers required treatment of metritis in another study.[3] Studies into induced parturition in cows show similar findings, with no RP cases needing treatment and no reported effect on subsequent fertility in these cows.[44,48] When evaluating the prophylactic use of long-acting oxytetracycline, it was determined that this method effectively reduced treatment rates in heifers aborted during the first and second trimester but increased the total cost of antimicrobial therapy to a point that it would not be cost-effective given the cost of long-acting oxytetracycline at the time the study was conducted.[2] However, long-acting oxytetracycline prices have reduced significantly since the time of study (authors' observations).

The exact mechanisms involved in the development of RP has yet to be fully established. It has been postulated that the frequency of RP in cattle aborted with dexamethasone is caused by a lower-than-normal estrogen spike at parturition.[43] However, the addition of exogenous estrogens to a parturition-induction protocol was not successful in decreasing the frequency of RP.[43] Maturation of the placenta and immune response against the fetal membranes have received much attention, and it has been widely established that these factors play a role in the occurrence of RP.[59–63] It is hypothesized that induced parturition interferes with proper maturation of the placenta, thus hindering the immune-assisted detachment of the fetal membranes.[59]

Fetal mummification has also been associated with pharmaceutical induction of abortion in heifers as a possible consequence. When aborting heifers at 4 to 6 months and 6 to 8 months, fetal mummies occurred at a rate of 2 per 40 in both groups, respectively.[27] The factors responsible for the development of fetal mummification are poorly understood.[27,64] Treatment of mummified fetuses can be accomplished through additional dosing of prostaglandins and in some cases manual assistance to remove the fetus from the vagina.[34–39,65]

In addition, the potential stress of induced abortions along with the use of dexamethasone as an abortifacient can impair immune function, potentially making these animals more susceptible to other diseases, such as bovine respiratory disease

(BRD).[1,66] The immunosuppressive effects of dexamethasone are intricate, and the effects on specific cell populations are variable. Lymphopenia and neutrophilia are common findings in cattle administered dexamethasone.[67–70] Certain populations of lymphocytes are more susceptible to the effects of dexamethasone[67,71–73] and may undergo drug-induced apoptosis[72] or reduced function.[70,72,74] There are also many alterations in the expression of multiple cell surface receptors[67,69] and the production of cytokines.[73,74] The increase in neutrophils is characterized by a transient mature neutrophilia caused by the release of marginated neutrophils.[68] Although an increase in the number of circulating neutrophils is observed, it has been shown that neutrophil migration into tissues is likely impaired[68] as well as the functional abilities of these neutrophils.[74,75] Dexamethasone also alters the expression of immune peptides in respiratory tract secretions.[76,77]

It has been postulated that antiinflammatory drugs, of which dexamethasone would be in the steroidal antiinflammatory class, may be of benefit in modulating the immune-related damage associated with BRD.[78,79] However, studies into the effect of dexamethasone treatment on the clinical progression of BRD are inconclusive because of design limitations.[80] The current body of knowledge suggests that the immunosuppressive consequences associated with dexamethasone administration likely outweigh any benefits it may provide,[81–84] but no definitive conclusions can be made at this time.[80,85] Dexamethasone administered to induce abortion in feedlot heifers should be done so with full consideration of the immunosuppressive effects to ensure management steps are in place to reduce or control the risk of BRD.

It is well documented that dairy cows undergo an immunosuppressive state during the periparturient period characterized primarily by impaired leukocyte function[86–88] and changes in specific leukocyte populations (primarily T cell populations).[89,90] This state has partially been attributed to the physiologic stress of lactation; however, many hormonal and neuroendocrine changes occur during this period that may influence cytokine production and negatively affect leukocyte migration and function.[86] Although there are likely breed effects as well as differences between natural parturition and induced abortion, one may postulate that the physiologic stress of aborting heifers has immunosuppressive consequences in addition to the administration of exogenous corticosteroids as mentioned previously.

Because of the concerns of further immunosuppression in heifers deemed at high risk of developing BRD, it is sometimes elected to postpone induction of abortion, especially when dexamethasone is to be used. It may be warranted to delay abortion until approximately 21 days after arrival if feasible, especially if these can be timed to coincide with other procedures, such as delayed implant or revaccination where applicable.[1,20]

Although there is currently nothing published on the public perception regarding pregnant heifer management, it is imperative that these factors be considered. Increased rate of dystocia and calving complications are inevitable when heifers reach parturition during the feeding period. Live calves that are born in a feedlot setting are introduced into an environment that does not bode well for proper development and immune function. These complications can be greatly reduced by appropriate arrival protocols to reduce the number of heifers that deliver calves while on feed; therefore, abortion may be seen as a humane option. However, the need to abort heifers in the first place not only creates economic constraints for the producer but it may also be seen as inappropriate by the general public. Therefore, it is important that as an industry we try to move toward a system in which few or no pregnant heifers are placed on feed to begin with.

HUMAN HEALTH CONCERNS

The use of prostaglandins, such as cloprostenol sodium and dinoprost tromethamine, poses serious potential health risks to humans. Those of most concern are miscarriages and bronchospasm. These products are readily absorbed through the skin; therefore, waterproof gloves must be worn at all times, and women of childbearing age or asthmatic individuals should not handle these products. In the case that these products do come in contact with skin, the area should be immediately cleansed with soap and water. If these products come in contact with eyes, they should be flushed under running water for 15 minutes. Respiratory emergencies that may occur can often be controlled through the administration of a rapidly absorbed bronchodilator. In the case of inadvertent exposure, immediate attention of a health professional is advisable (present package insert or Material Safety Data Sheet (MSDS) information if seeking medical help).[32–39,91]

SUMMARY

Although the ideal situation would be to not feed any pregnant heifers, decreased feeder supplies make this option impractical in many instances. Pregnant heifers in the feedlot represent a substantial economic liability to the cattle feeder because of the decreased feed efficiency on a carcass-adjusted basis, decreased slaughter value, and increased death losses and health costs.[1,3,4,7,12,13] Complications and adverse outcomes associated with parturition pose many challenges for the feedlot and can lead to decreased employee morale (authors' observations).[3,13,46]

Many strategies exist for managing pregnant heifers on feedlot arrival, or shortly thereafter, to decrease the economic losses associated with feeding pregnant heifers.[1,7,12,13] Although there are some situations in which nothing is done to manage pregnant heifers entering the feedlot, the mainstay of many management strategies is the use of abortifacients to terminate pregnancies early in the feeding period.[11] The effectiveness of abortifacient strategies will vary based on the stage of gestation; as a result, the pharmacologic approach to termination of pregnancy depends on the stage of gestation.[3,24,25,27,48] When using pharmaceuticals, particularly prostaglandins, to abort heifers, every precaution must be taken to reduce the risk of human exposure. Those at risk of more serious consequences (eg, women and asthmatic individuals) should not handle these products, and appropriate care must be taken to reduce the risk of inadvertent exposure.[32–39,91]

In order to make economically sound management decisions, the feedlot should be aware of the economic liabilities associated with pregnant heifers so that they can make informed purchases and appropriate management decisions. These strategies may be determined at the individual animal level based on the results of various pregnancy diagnosis options or at a group level based on historical experience and expected stage of gestation for each group of heifers. Expected pregnancy risk on a group basis is fundamental in determining the most economical management strategy.[13] Regardless of the strategy implemented, it is important to understand that when purchase price for the same weight heifers is equivalent, aborting heifers will result in lower returns than feeding heifers that were never pregnant to start with.[3,12,13]

REFERENCES

1. MacGregor S, Falkner T, Stokka G. Managing pregnant heifers in the feedlot. Compendium on Continuing Education for the Practicing Veterinarian (USA) 1997;19:1389–407.

2. Booker CW, Jim GK, Guichon PT. A field trial to determine the efficacy of long-acting oxytetracycline for reducing the treatment rate in aborted feedlot heifers. Can Vet J 1992;33:397–9.
3. Jim GK, Ribble CS, Guichon PT, et al. The relative economics of feeding open, aborted, pregnant feedlot heifers. Can Vet J 1991;32:613–7.
4. Stanton T, Birkelo C, Bennett B, et al. Effect of abortion on individually fed finishing heifer performance. Agri-Pract 1988;9:15–7.
5. Bennett BW, Clayton RP, Cravens RL, et al. Slaughter weight loss attributable to pregnancy in feedlot heifers. Mod Vet Pract 1984;65:677–9.
6. Clayton P, Lloyd B. Cost to the packer. In: Proceedings of the Academy of Veterinary Consultants. 1984. p. 28–43.
7. Edwards AJ, Laudert SB. Economic evaluation of the use of feedlot abortifacients. Bov Pract 1984;19:148–50.
8. Bishop G, Brethour J, Marston T, et al. Effects of pregnancy in feedlot heifers on performance and carcass characteristics. In: Conference papers of Cattlemen's Day. Manhattan (KS): 2003. p. 72–4.
9. Kreikemeier KK, Unruh JA. Carcass traits and the occurrence of dark cutters in pregnant and nonpregnant feedlot heifers. J Anim Sci 1993;71:1699–703.
10. Laudert SB. Incidence of pregnancy in feedlot heifers at slaughter. In: Conference papers of Cattlemen's Day. Manhattan (KS): 1988. p. 112–4.
11. USDA. Feedlot 2011 "Part I: management practices on U.S. feedlots with a capacity of 1,000 or more head." USDA–APHIS–VS–CEAH–NAHMS. Fort Collins (CO). #626.0313.
12. Bennett B. Economic liability: the pregnant feedlot heifer. Anim Nutr Health 1985; 40:5–8.
13. Buhman MJ, Hungerford LL, Smith DR. An economic risk assessment of the management of pregnant feedlot heifers in the USA. Prev Vet Med 2003;59:207–22.
14. Youngquist RS. Pregnancy diagnosis. In: Youngquist RS, Threlfall WR, editors. Current therapy in large animal theriogenology. 2nd edition. St Louis (MO): W.B. Saunders; 2007. p. 294–303.
15. Warnick LD, Mohammed HO, White ME, et al. The relationship of the interval from breeding to uterine palpation for pregnancy diagnosis with calving outcomes in Holstein cows. Theriogenology 1995;44:811–25.
16. Fricke PM, Lamb GC. Potential applications and pitfalls of reproductive ultrasonography in bovine practice. Vet Clin North Am Food Anim Pract 2005;21:419–36.
17. Pierson RA, Ginther OJ. Ultrasonography for detection of pregnancy and study of embryonic development in heifers. Theriogenology 1984;22:225–33.
18. Badtram GA, Gaines JD, Thomas CB, et al. Factors influencing the accuracy of early pregnancy detection in cattle by real-time ultrasound scanning of the uterus. Theriogenology 1991;35:1153–67.
19. Kastelic JP, Curran S, Ginther OJ. Accuracy of ultrasonography for pregnancy diagnosis on days 10 to 22 in heifers. Theriogenology 1989;31:813–20.
20. Bronson A, Edwards T. Management of pregnant heifers in the feedlot. In: Proceedings of the Academy of Veterinary Consultants. Calgary (Canada): 2008. p. 27–38.
21. Schafer DW. New technologies in the beef business. In: Proceedings of the Cattlemen's College, Arizona Cattlemen's Association Convention. Chandler (AZ): 2013. p. 11–4.
22. BioTracking. BioPRYN FAQs. BioTracking, LLC. Available at: http://www.biotracking.com/beef/biopryn/faqs. Accessed December 29, 2014.

23. IDEXX Laboratories. Bovine pregnancy. IDEXX Laboratories, Inc. Available at: https://www.idexx.com/livestock-poultry/ruminant/lpd-bovine-pregnancy-test.html. Accessed December 29, 2014.

24. Copeland DD, Schultz RH, Kemtrup ME. Induction of abortion in feedlot heifers with cloprostenol (a synthetic analogue of prostaglandin f2alpha): a dose response study. Can Vet J 1978;19:29–32.

25. Day AM. Cloprostenol for termination of pregnancy in cattle. B) The induction of abortion. N Z Vet J 1977;25:139–44.

26. McAllister JF, Lauderdale JW. Lutalyse in pregnancy termination. In: Proceedings of the Lutalyse Symposium. Brook Lodge: Augusta (MI); 1979. p. 65–74.

27. Barth AD, Adams WM, Manns JG, et al. Induction of abortion in feedlot heifers with a combination of cloprostenol and dexamethasone. Can Vet J 1981;22:62–4.

28. McDonald LE, Nichols RE, McNutt SH. Studies on corpus luteum ablation and progesterone replacement therapy during pregnancy in the cow. Am J Vet Res 1952;13:446–51.

29. Thomas PG. Induced abortion. In: Youngquist RS, Threlfall WR, editors. Current therapy in large animal theriogenology. 2nd edition. St Louis (MO): W.B. Saunders; 2007. p. 307–10.

30. Erb RE, Gomes WR, Randel RD, et al. Effect of ovariectomy on concentration of progesterone in blood plasma and urinary estrogen excretion rate in the pregnant bovine. J Dairy Sci 1968;51:420–7.

31. Wendorf GL, Lawyer MS, First NL. Role of the adrenals in the maintenance of pregnancy in cows. J Reprod Fertil 1983;68:281–7.

32. Lutalyse, Zoetis Canada. North American Compendiums, Ltd. Canada. 2014. Available at: http://cca.naccvp.com/product/view/1198298. Accessed December 29, 2014.

33. Lutalyse Injection, Zoetis Inc. North American Compendiums, Inc. United States. 2014. Available at: http://bayerall.naccvp.com/product/view/3690361. Accessed December 29, 2014.

34. estroPLAN, Parnell U.S. 1, Inc. North American Compendiums, Inc. United States. 2014. Available at: http://bayerall.naccvp.com/product/view/1665000. Accessed December 29, 2014.

35. Estrumate, Merck. Animal Health, Intervet Canada Corp. North American Compendiums, Ltd. Canada. 2014. Available at: http://cca.naccvp.com/product/view/1208034. Accessed December 29, 2014.

36. Estrumate, Merck. Animal Health, Intervet Inc. North American Compendiums, Inc. United States. 2014. Available at: http://bayerall.naccvp.com/product/view/1047067. Accessed December 29, 2014.

37. Juramate, Bimeda-MTC Animal Health Inc. North American Compendiums, Ltd. Canada. 2014. Available at: http://cca.naccvp.com/product/view/1473005. Accessed December 29, 2014.

38. estroPLAN injection, Vétoquinol N.-A. Inc. North American Compendiums, Ltd. Canada. 2014. Available at: http://cca.naccvp.com/product/view/1234317?key=label. Accessed December 29, 2014.

39. Cloprostenol Veyx, Modern Veterinary Therapeutics, LLC. North American Compendiums, Ltd. Canada. 2014. Available at: http://cca.naccvp.com/product/view/1354008. Accessed December 29, 2014.

40. Henricks DM, Rawlings NC, Ellicott AR, et al. Use of prostaglandin f2alpha to induce parturition in beef heifers. J Anim Sci 1977;44:438–41.

41. Adams WM, Wagner WC. The role of corticoids in parturition. Biol Reprod 1970;3:223–8.

42. Welch R, Newling P, Anderson D. Induction of parturition in cattle with corticosteroids: an analysis of field trials. N Z Vet J 1973;21:103–8.
43. Barth AD, Adams WM, Manns JC, et al. Induction of parturition in beef cattle using estrogens in conjunction with dexamethasone. Can Vet J 1978;19:175–80.
44. Lauderdale JW. Effect of corticoid administration in bovine pregnancy. J Am Vet Med Assoc 1972;160:867–71.
45. Bosc MJ, Fevre J, Vaslet De Fontaubert Y. A comparison of induction of parturition with dexamethasone or with an analog of prostaglandin f2α (a-pgf) in cattle. Theriogenology 1975;3:187–91.
46. Johnson WH, Manns JG, Adams WM, et al. Termination of pregnancy with cloprostenol and dexamethasone in intact or ovariectomized cows. Can Vet J 1981;22:288–90.
47. Terrell SP, Thomson DU, Wileman BW, et al. A survey to describe current feeder cattle health and well-being program recommendations made by feedlot veterinary consultants in the united states and Canada. Bov Pract 2011;45: 140–8.
48. Lewing FJ, Proulx J, Mapletoft RJ. Induction of parturition in the cow using cloprostenol and dexamethasone in combination. Can Vet J 1985;26:317–22.
49. MGA 100 PREMIX, Zoetis Canada. North American Compendiums, Ltd. Canada. 2014. Available at: http://cca.naccvp.com/product/view/1198299. Accessed December 29, 2014.
50. MGA 200 PREMIX, Zoetis Inc. North American Compendiums, Inc. United States. 2014. Available at: http://bayerall.naccvp.com/product/view/1049032. Accessed December 29, 2014.
51. Bloss R, Northam J, Smith L, et al. Effects of oral melengestrol acetate on the performance of feedlot cattle. J Anim Sci 1966;25:1048–53.
52. Horstman LA, Callahan CJ, Morter RL, et al. Ovariectomy as a means of abortion and control of estrus in feedlot heifers. Theriogenology 1982;17:273–92.
53. Perrett T, Wildman BK, Jim GK, et al. Evaluation of the efficacy and cost-effectiveness of melengestrol acetate in feedlot heifer calves in western Canada. Vet Ther 2008;9:223–40.
54. Sides G, Vasconcelos J, Borg R, et al. A comparison of melengestrol acetate fed at two dose levels to feedlot heifers. The Professional Animal Scientist 2009;25: 731–6.
55. Wagner J, Davis N, Reinhardt C. A meta-analysis evaluation of feeding melengestrol acetate to feedlot heifers implanted with estradiol, trenbolone acetate, or the combination of estradiol and trenbolone acetate. The Professional Animal Scientist 2007;23:625–31.
56. Zimbelman RG, Smith LW. Maintenance of pregnancy in ovariectomized heifers with melengestrol acetate. J Anim Sci 1966;25:207–11.
57. Johnson K, Erb R. Maintenance of pregnancy in ovariectomized cattle with progestin compounds and their effect on progestin levels in the corpus luteum. J Dairy Sci 1962;45:633–9.
58. Allen J, Herring J. The induction of parturition using dexamethasone in dairy cattle. Aust Vet J 1976;52:442–5.
59. Benedictus L, Jorritsma R, Knijn HM, et al. Chemotactic activity of cotyledons for mononuclear leukocytes related to occurrence of retained placenta in dexamethasone induced parturition in cattle. Theriogenology 2011;76:802–9.
60. Boos A, Janssen V, Mulling C. Proliferation and apoptosis in bovine placentomes during pregnancy and around induced and spontaneous parturition as well as in cows retaining the fetal membranes. Reproduction 2003;126:469–80.

61. Davies CJ, Hill JR, Edwards JL, et al. Major histocompatibility antigen expression on the bovine placenta: its relationship to abnormal pregnancies and retained placenta. Anim Reprod Sci 2004;82/83:267–80.
62. Hartmann D, Bollwein H, Honnens A, et al. Protracted induction of parturition enhances placental maturation, but does not influence incidence of placental retention in cows. Theriogenology 2013;80:185–92.
63. Kamemori Y, Wakamiya K, Nishimura R, et al. Expressions of apoptosis-regulating factors in bovine retained placenta. Placenta 2011;32:20–6.
64. Drost M. Maternal and fetal disorders during gestation. In: Proceedings of the North American Veterinary Conference. Orlando (FL): 2011. p. 45–7.
65. Lefebvre RC, Saint-Hilaire E, Morin I, et al. Retrospective case study of fetal mummification in cows that did not respond to prostaglandin f2alpha treatment. Can Vet J 2009;50:71–6.
66. Ackermann MR, Derscheid R, Roth JA. Innate immunology of bovine respiratory disease. Vet Clin North Am Food Anim Pract 2010;26:215–28.
67. Anderson BH, Watson DL, Colditz IG. The effect of dexamethasone on some immunological parameters in cattle. Vet Res Commun 1999;23:399–413.
68. Burton JL, Kehrli ME, Kapil S, et al. Regulation of l-selectin and cd18 on bovine neutrophils by glucocorticoids: effects of cortisol and dexamethasone. J Leukoc Biol 1995;57:317–25.
69. Lan HC, Reddy PG, Chambers MA, et al. Effect of stress on interleukin-2 receptor expression by bovine mononuclear leukocytes. Vet Immunol Immunopathol 1995;49:241–9.
70. Pruett JH, Fisher WF, Deloach JR. Effects of dexamethasone on selected parameters of the bovine immune system. Vet Res Commun 1987;11:305–23.
71. Maslanka T. Effect of dexamethasone and meloxicam on counts of selected t lymphocyte subpopulations and NK cells in cattle - in vivo investigations. Res Vet Sci 2014;96:338–46.
72. Maslanka T, Jaroszewski JJ. In vitro effects of dexamethasone on bovine cd25+cd4+ and cd25-cd4+ cells. Res Vet Sci 2012;93:1367–79.
73. Menge C, Dean-Nystrom EA. Dexamethasone depletes gammadelta t cells and alters the activation state and responsiveness of bovine peripheral blood lymphocyte subpopulations. J Dairy Sci 2008;91:2284–98.
74. Ohmann HB, Baker PE, Babiuk LA. Effect of dexamethasone on bovine leukocyte functions and bovine herpesvirus type-1 replication. Can J Vet Res 1987;51:350–7.
75. Roth JA, Kaeberle ML. Effects of in vivo dexamethasone administration on in vitro bovine polymorphonuclear leukocyte function. Infect Immun 1981;33:434–41.
76. Mitchell GB, Al-Haddawi MH, Clark ME, et al. Effect of corticosteroids and neuropeptides on the expression of defensins in bovine tracheal epithelial cells. Infect Immun 2007;75:1325–34.
77. Mitchell GB, Clark ME, Caswell JL. Alterations in the bovine bronchoalveolar lavage proteome induced by dexamethasone. Vet Immunol Immunopathol 2007;118:283–93.
78. Malazdrewich C, Thumbikat P, Maheswaran SK. Protective effect of dexamethasone in experimental bovine pneumonic mannheimiosis. Microb Pathog 2004;36:227–36.
79. Moiré N, Roy O, Gardey L. Effects of dexamethasone on distribution and function of peripheral mononuclear blood cells in pneumonic calves. Vet Immunol Immunopathol 2002;87:459–66.

80. Francoz D, Buczinski S, Apley M. Evidence related to the use of ancillary drugs in bovine respiratory disease (anti-inflammatory and others): are they justified or not? Vet Clin North Am Food Anim Pract 2012;28:23–38.

81. Bureau F, Weerdt ML, Hanon E, et al. Control of inflammation in experimental bovine pneumonic pasteurellosis. Bov Pract 1998;32:5–13.

82. Chiang YW, Roth JA, Andrews JJ. Influence of recombinant bovine interferon γ and dexamethasone on pneumonia attributable to haemophilus somnus in calves. Am J Vet Res 1990;51:759–62.

83. Christie BM, Pierson RE, Braddy PM, et al. Efficacy of corticosteroids as supportive therapy for bronchial pneumonia in yearling feedlot cattle. Bov Pract 1977;12: 115–7.

84. Davies DH, Duncan JR. The pathogenesis of recurrent infections with infectious bovine rhinotracheitis virus induced in calves by treatment with corticosteroids. Cornell Vet 1974;64:340–66.

85. Fajt V, Lechtenberg K. Using anti-inflammatories in the treatment of bovine respiratory disease. Large Animal Practice 1998;34(6):8–9.

86. Kehrli ME Jr, Kimura K, Goff JP, et al. Immunological dysfunction in periparturient cows - what role does it play in postpartum infectious diseases? In: Proceedings of the Thirty-Second Annual Conference American Association of Bovine Practitioners. Nashville (TN): 1999. p. 24–8.

87. Kehrli ME Jr, Nonnecke BJ, Roth JA. Alterations in bovine lymphocyte function during the periparturient period. Am J Vet Res 1989;50:215–20.

88. Kehrli ME Jr, Nonnecke BJ, Roth JA. Alterations in bovine neutrophil function during the periparturient period. Am J Vet Res 1989;50:207–14.

89. Kimura K, Goff JP, Kehrli ME Jr, et al. Phenotype analysis of peripheral blood mononuclear cells in periparturient dairy cows. J Dairy Sci 1999;82:315–9.

90. Van Kampen C, Mallard BA. Effects of peripartum stress and health on circulating bovine lymphocyte subsets. Vet Immunol Immunopathol 1997;59:79–91.

91. Lust EB, Barthold C, Malesker MA, et al. Human health hazards of veterinary medications: information for emergency departments. J Emerg Med 2011;40: 198–207.

Current Status of Parasite Control at the Feed Yard

Thomas A. Yazwinski, PhD*, Chris A. Tucker, PhD, Jeremy Powell, PhD, DVM, Paul Beck, PhD, Eva Wray, BS, Christine Weingartz, BS

KEYWORDS

- Feedlot cattle • Parasites • Anthelmintics • Nematodes • Receiving

KEY POINTS

- Fly and louse infestations are readily discerned and remedied in feedlot cattle.
- Tapeworm and fluke infections are accepted as probable but, given the lack of anthelmintics with realistic efficacy against these infections, these helminths are allowed to persist without treatment.
- Nematode infections are considered ubiquitous with cattle coming from pasture and are targeted with a macrocyclic lactone (ML), usually in combination with a benzimidazole.
- Populations of nematodes seem to be effectively controlled by a combination of anthelmintic treatment, animal resistance and resilience, lack of reinfection, and diet.

Producer-perceived importance of parasitisms in the beef industry is most elevated at the stocker level, of lesser gravity at the cow-calf level, and of least significance at the feed yard. The reduced perceived importance at the feed yard is contingent on the administration of an anthelmintic (alone or in combination with a complementary anthelmintic) at receiving and insecticidal remedies put in place when warranted. To that point, it has been aptly stated, "stocker operations provide a large proportion of the health and nutritional management of young, lightweight animals that feedlots prefer to avoid when possible."[1] At the feed yard, parasite significance is dwarfed by the consideration directed toward economics (animal and feed), supply (animal and feed), the 24/7 management of animals, facilities and waste, and, finally, oversight and control of microbial and viral diseases (primarily respiratory). More attention is provided at the feed yard for fly (stable and face) and pest bird (starling) control than to the possible postarrival presence and importance of parasites. Only a visit to a feed yard is needed to achieve this mind-set. The animals are in exceptional condition, under constant monitoring for health and appetite, and fed extensively researched diets at prescribed rates—a system of production that seems to cancel

The authors have nothing to disclose.
Department of Animal Sciences, University of Arkansas, B110D, Fayetteville, AR 72701, USA
* Corresponding author.
E-mail address: yazwinsk@uark.edu

Vet Clin Food Anim 31 (2015) 229–245
http://dx.doi.org/10.1016/j.cvfa.2015.03.005
0749-0720/15/$ – see front matter Published by Elsevier Inc.

vetfood.theclinics.com

(or conceal) any direct or indirect cause of economic impact due to parasites. Given these conditions, there is still much to be cited relative to parasite control at the feed yard: the parasites, the parasiticides, and animal performance/productivity given the interplay of the two and what needs to be done in the future relative to parasite control and assessment at the feed yard.

QUESTIONNAIRE QUESTIONS AND ANSWERS

In writing an article about controlling parasitisms of feedlot cattle, information should be included as provided by the people who actually oversee the cattle and whatever management and treatment are prescribed for parasite control. To that end, a questionnaire was circulated to 10 feedlot veterinarians who are collectively responsible for monitoring millions of feedlot cattle for disease prevention; and millions of cattle that are replaced by millions more approximately every 4 months. Unfortunately, only 4 sets of answers were received that were comprehensive. From many face-to-face discussions with these veterinarians and their peers, the authors think that the limited answers did accurately portray the appreciation for parasites at the feed yard and those actions (as well as mind-sets) that result. A fifth veterinarian confided that the answers to these questions are to some degree "corporate property"—the results of many experiences, in-house studies, corporate round tables, and so forth. The authors appreciate this opinion. Having said that, the authors thank the respondents—feedlot veterinarians, who, for the sake of their anonymity, are quoted as veterinarians a, b, c, and d. The questions and their answers follow.

Question 1: Are lice the only external parasites to consider when treating incoming cattle?

a. Lice during the winter are our target pest. Grubs are rare but costly due to carcass trim. We use Cydectin, Dectomax, or Ivomec for worm control and get grubs as a freebie. We treat all cattle for lice starting in October and ending in March with a pour-on pyrethrin at initial processing and again at reimplant. If we have a "lice break" during the feeding period, we will mist (fog) the cattle at the feed bunk to avoid running them through the chute again.
   Stable flies are a big problem for cattle at the perimeter of the pens. Seems like the flies are too lazy to fly deep into the feedlot, attacking the first cattle they find. Parasitic wasps are commonly used for control along with manure management, cleaning up forage debris and mowing grass around the feedlots to less than 4 inches. Ticks, horn flies, and face flies are not a problem, and house flies pester people more than the cattle.

b. Louse infestations are the only externals we consider important on cattle at arrival. We use injectable ivermectin year round for worms, and we feel that gets the sucking lice. From November to March, we also use a pour-on permethrin. Cattle coming into the southern yards don't get the pour-on, because we don't see large lice burdens on those cattle.
   We use premise spray and bait for house flies and parasitic wasps for stable flies. Pen maintenance and minimizing standing water and manure is also a focal point for controlling flies.
   Where we get into issues with flies is when we get abnormally wet weather during optimal fly temperatures. Our approach in that case is more of the same: pen maintenance and aggressive premise spraying.

c. Lice are the big problem, but we still see grubs. We start using pyrethrin pour-on around October 1, and continue to spring. If we get long periods of overcast and

cold weather, the lice seem to persist. We use parasitoids and fogging for stable and house flies. Stable flies can be a real problem certain times of the years regardless of what you do.
d. All incoming cattle are treated with topical ivermectin (in combination with fenbendazole), and the ivermectin generally takes care of any lice. Any pediculosis during the feeding phase is dealt with on a per-pen basis with a pour-on pyrethroid.

Question 2: Are cocci a problem at the feed yard?
a. Coccidiosis not much of a problem. We use an ionophore in most of our early rations (exception is "natural" beef), and that seems to control cocci. I do see severe coccidiosis in cattle coming in from Mexico. If we have clinical coccidiosis in our new cattle, we give them amprolium. Feedlot conditions don't seem to favor development of coccidiosis; animals generally have it or not when they come.
b. Occasionally, we see coccidiosis outbreaks and we deal with it on a pen-by-pen basis. I feel that getting new cattle on an ionophore as soon as possible controls the cocci along with improving feed efficiency [FE]. Along with monensin, we have used amprolium and decoquinate. When we do get clinical coccidiosis, it will be tied to a failure to include monensin in the ration, along with real bad wet and muddy conditions. We don't float feces for cocci to confirm the condition but rather go with predisposing history, diarrhea, hematochezia, neurologic signs, and mortality.
c. Looks like coccidiosis is mainly controlled with monensin in the diets. Occasionally, with "natural" cattle, we'll get coccidiosis as evidenced by bloody stools and high oocyst counts.
d. Coccidiosis is generally not a problem, but if we do get it, we use amprolium.

Question 3: Do you ever perplex over which worms are arriving with your cattle: flukes versus tapes versus roundworms?
a. We don't fret over flukes or tapes. Our concerns are *Ostertagia* and *Cooperia*.
b. It does perplex me. We receive cattle from all over the country as well as from out of the country. Additionally, we coincidentally feed numerous classes of cattle. Therefore, we have elected to go with the KISS procedure (keep it simple stupid) and base our decisions on in-house, well replicated, and randomized studies.
c. Perplex on it every day.
d. Not perplexed. All new cattle get ivermectin pour-on and oral fenbendazole. Case closed!

Question 4: How about tapeworms: intestinal tapes as well as measeled meat?
a. Meat measles are a concern. Had one animal positive about 5 years ago and the US Department of Agriculture as well as state investigators got involved immediately! Several years before that, I remember an outbreak in Texas that was precipitated by a sewage plant malfunction resulting in contaminated cottonseed hulls that eventually went into cattle feed distributed to 3 states!
Sporadic outbreaks are probably due to improper toilet practices by infected people. Measles is uncommon now, due mostly to improper personal habits. As to recent problems with measeled meat, seems like there's been some in the Pacific Northwest involving contaminated potato waste getting into cattle feed.
b. Not aware of any problems with measly meat. I'm sure the packing plants would let us know if we had it, and I haven't heard anything in years.

c. Haven't seen any *Cysticercus bovis* in years. In recent years, it's been in the Northwest and associated with potato waste.

Question 5: How about flukes? Do you ascertain if cattle are coming from "fluky" country and then use a flukicide if flukes are to be expected?
a. Damage from flukes is done when we get the cattle, so we don't address them.
b. We do a decent job of knowing what part of the country cattle are coming from, and cattle from fluky country (Gulf Coast states and Pacific Northwest) get a flukicide (clorsulon). However, I have strong reservations that this does any good.
c. Difficult to ascertain. We do not routinely use flukicides because of lack of effectiveness.
d. Do not routinely use a flukicide at this time.

Question 6: For nematodes, what is your current receiving treatment regime: drugs, combinations, repeated treatments, formulations, and so forth?
a. No pour-ons or generics. I prefer moxidectin, but if a client is married to the doramectin or ivermectin salesperson, I recommend combination deworming. We only deworm at initial processing. Treat everyone based on average weight rounded up to the next 100 pounds.
b. Our non-Holsteins get injectable, generic ivermectin combined with fenbendazole at initial processing. We treat based on each animal's bodyweight. Holsteins don't get anything. They are coming from confinement feeding and are clean.
c. Injectable pioneer ivermectin plus a white wormer, at receiving, based on average pay weights.
d. All arriving cattle get ivermectin pour-on combined with oral fenbendazole. All cattle treated at average truck load weight.

Question 7: Do you feel there's a difference in effectives: ML versus ML, benzimidazole versus benzimidazole, generic versus pioneer, and so forth?
a. Prefer pioneer and prefer moxidectin. For benzimidazoles, I recommend fenbendazole or oxfendazole, no preference.
b. Based on our in-house work, there are minimal differences between injectable ivermectins, so generic ivermectin is our drug of choice. As for the benzimidazoles, we treat them as commodities and consider dose volume and pricing. I do worry about post-treatment product loss with the drenches.
c. We use moxidectin with fenbendazole. They have the best data behind them.
d. Don't feel there is that much difference between the anthelmintics.

Question 8: Is worm resistance a problem at the feed yard?
a. There's resistance on the farm and ranches, so of course there's resistance at the feed yard. I'm looking into doing fecal egg count reduction (FECR) tests in the future to spot check.
b. Hard to say. We have very good cattle performance (average daily gain [ADG] and feed conversions), so that makes me wonder if it's a big issue. We are concerned about the use of certain products in the stocker industry (eg, long-range eprinomectin) and how that will impact resistance and cattle feeding. So far, we've been relying on FECR tests conducted by pharmaceutical reps (bias??).
c. I think resistance is a problem on occasion. We haven't checked on our drug effectiveness in years.
d. Yes, there is a resistance problem.

Question 9: Do you feel confident that worms are not a problem at the feedlot once the animals are dewormed at arrival (ie, drug[s] worked well and no new infections are acquired during the feedlot phase)?

a. Don't see a problem with worms in our feedlot cattle. Also, we use injectable MLs at label dose or higher, and that should get arrested *Ostertagia*.

b. We do hit the cattle hard with a combination at receiving to "clean" them out. I don't expect any reinfection, so unless resistance is a real issue (doesn't seem to be a big problem), I don't see any issues, and that's with doing a fair number of necropsies. Also, don't see any problems with arrested *Ostertagia*, and that's after a large, in-house study.

c. Don't think worms are a problem at the feed yard, may be mistaken. I do worry about arrested *Ostertagia*.

d. Worms, including arrested *Ostertagia*, are not a problem at feed yard.

Question 10: Why are you using your current anthelmintic(s)? Effectiveness? Price? Supplier?

a. We base our decision on published data.

b. All of these. Also, we conduct in-house work on (1) animal biological response, (2) cost of that response, and (3) administration issues. There's also supplier reputation and service.

c. The owners decide on the anthelmintic that is used. Usually, it's pricing and the result of "bundling" programs.

d. We check our anthelmintic efficacies with the FECR test.

Question 11: Do you feel certain breeds/sexes translate into different parasitisms?

a. Don't know if breed or sex translates into different parasite problems. Animal history definitely does, but we don't get the history of parasite treatments. We handle all animals the same because they come mixed from various auctions and clients. We simply can't track them.

b. Don't know about sex, but if it is then it's pretty low on the list of factors. For breeds, the northern-type, longer haired cattle (*Bos taurus*) do have more louse problems than the *Bos indicus* cattle. Geographic source and animal history are the top factors contributing to parasitisms. For instance, cattle that come from dry areas or confined feeding programs (our Holsteins) and cold places (Canada) have low worm burdens.

c. Don't know if breed or sex factors into parasite levels.

d. Animal breed or sex does not translate into variations in parasitisms.

Question 12: Do you feel worms are important relative to the effectiveness of vaccines and antibiotics at the feed yard?

a. Yes! I feel that we have more death losses today at the feed yard than when I graduated from vet school many years ago. Anything that is immunosuppressive (eg, worms) results in increased antibiotic usage, death loss, and economic loss.

b. Wish I had the answer to this! Overall, my answer is yes. The research I'm familiar with shows that heavy worm burdens decrease vaccine response, increase predisposition to disease, decrease overall response to antibiotics, and hamper the animal's fight against disease. What level of parasitism that is, I don't know. A parasite dose titration study would be interesting!

c. Probably not.

d. No evidence to suggest there is an issue with worms and vaccine/antibiotic effectiveness. In any case, we eliminate all parasites at receiving.

Question 13: What else should be mentioned relative to parasites and feed yards?
a. We need more clinical work at the feed yard to better define the parasite control practices that translate into economic return!
b. Looks like you covered it. But I might mention, I have witnessed bias by the pharmaceutical industry (or their parasitologists) when it comes to reading fecal samples. Gives me strong reservations about whose findings are valid and whose are not.
c. Nothing I can think of. But, we need a better solution for these stable fly populations! Last summer (2013) was real bad!
d. Nothing else.

DISCUSSION

For the sake of congruity, this discussion follows the same sequence of subject matter as the previous questionnaire. In addition, **Table 1** provides a list of the parasites most likely to have a presence at the feed yard, presented by taxonomic classification and probable potential for significance at the feed yard.

The Ectoparasites

The external parasites of importance at the feed yard are the lice (sucking and biting) and flies (stable). Judging from the questionnaire answers, myiasis by *Hypoderma* spp

Table 1
Common parasites with the potential to impact animal performance at the feed yard

Category	Scientific Name	Common Name	Likelihood of Impact
Nematode	*Ostertagia ostertagi*	Brown stomach worm	High
	Haemonchus placei	Barber pole worm	High
	Oesophagostomum radiatum	Nodular worm	High
	Cooperia punctata	Cooperiad	High
Trematode	*Fasciola hepatica*	Liver fluke	High
Insect	*Stomoxys calcitrans*	Stable fly	High
Nematode	*C oncophora*	Cooperiad	Moderate
Cestode	*Moniezia benedeni*	Tapeworm	Moderate
Insect	*Bovicola (Damalinia) bovis*	Biting louse	Moderate
	Linognathus vituli	Long-nose sucking louse	Moderate
Nematode	*Nematodirus helvetianus*	Thread-necked worm	Low
	Strongyloides papillosus	Threadworm	Low
	Bunostomum phlebotomum	Hookworm	Low
	Trichostrongylus axei	Small stomach worm	Low
	C spatulata	Cooperiad	Low
	C pectinata	Cooperiad	Low
	Dictyocaulus viviparus	Lungworm	Low
	Trichuris spp	Whipworm	Low
Trematode	*Fascioloides magna*	Deer fluke	Low
Cestode	*Cysticercus bovis (Taenia saginata)*	Bladder worm	Low
Insect	*Solenopotes capillatus*	Little blue louse	Low
	Haematopinus eurysternus	Short-nose sucking louse	Low
	Hypoderma lineatum	Common cattle grub	Low
	H bovis	Northern cattle grub	Low
Protozoa	*Eimeria* spp	Cocci	Low

seems to be all but totally dismissed from the radar at the feed yard. To illustrate the decline of grub infections (myiasis) in cattle, when ivermectin first became commercially available in the United States (1982), a major precondition for its use late in the grazing season was prior treatment of the cattle with a systemic insecticide so that the migrating instars would not be in an anatomic location to cause untoward effects when the ML was used (esophagitis and bloat with *Hypoderma lineatum* and posterior paralysis with *H bovis*). Now, *Hypoderma* spp infections are uncommon. Indicative of the low prevalence of grubs today, when a feed yard manager was asked how much "warble" he sees, his answer was, "What's a warble?" Mange mite (psoroptic and chorioptic) infestations, and the dipping vats they once necessitated, also seem relegated to the history book in North America. Face and horn flies are also of little significance at the feed yard, generally considered of consequence for grazing animals only.

Pediculosis, primarily due to the biting louse (*Bovicola bovis*) and the long-nose sucking louse (*Linognathus vituli*), is a seasonal condition and addressed at the feed yards from fall to spring. Topically applied insecticides, usually pyrethroids, are used by many for lice. MLs are also effective, but efficacies are extremely varied (biting louse vs sucking louse, ML vs ML, and injectable ML vs topical ML). Given the normal route of louse transmission (animal-to-animal contact), feedlot housing makes it mandatory that pediculosis be addressed proactively during favorable conditions (fall to spring).

Stable flies (*Stomoxys calcitrans*) are persistent, attacking, hematophagic ectoparasites that require control at all feed yards when temperatures are above freezing. These controls include (1) the routine removal of decaying organic debris used by the fly for immature stage development (egg to pupa), (2) insecticide application directly onto the cattle to kill the adult flies, and (3) parasitoid use. The insecticides used are primarily pyrethroids. The parasitic wasps (*Muscidifurax, Spalangia,* and *Nasonia* spp) are obtained commercially at the pupal stage and placed as well as subsequently managed at the feed yard for the entire fly season.[2] These biological controls for stable flies also aid in the control of house flies. Relative to the maintenance of effective parasitoid populations at the feed yard, the common if not universal use of ML endectocides at receiving might have a negative impact, because these highly potent and environmentally persistent compounds have been documented to elicit detrimental effects on nontarget arthropods, including parasitoids.[3]

Coccidiosis

Eimeria spp are the only protozoa addressed in this article and the only protozoa considered relevant by the veterinarians who answered the questionnaire. Trichomoniasis, cryptosporidiosis, giardiasis, neosporosis, and toxoplasmosis are all extremely important protozoan diseases that affect various phases of the cattle industry but, thankfully, are not of concern at the feed yard.

Intestinal coccidiosis of cattle is due to approximately 12 different species of *Eimeria*.[4] Well documented in a recent article,[5] coccidiosis is most pronounced in young cattle, with a combination of adequate exposure and predisposing factors (stress, lack of immunity, challenge, and so forth) resulting in heavy infections early in an animal's life subsequently giving way to light infections by a limited number of species. *Eimeria bovis* appears to be the predominate species in the United States. Generally, once animals arrive at the feed yard, they are already fairly immune to reinfection. Additionally, ionophore-containing diets, common at the feed yard, curtail endogenous development of *Eimeria* spp. This scenario relative to intestinal coccidiosis at the feed yard might continue to hold true in the future. At the current time, however, there is a vacuum in the supply of cattle to the feed yard, the result of previous drought conditions across the United States, low cow-calf numbers, and never-before-seen prices per pound at the grocery store. Due to the economic impetus for keeping the feed yards full, lighter weight and/or younger cattle are being delivered, animals that would inherently be of greater disease risk coincident with reduced effectiveness of chemical intervention, such as with coccidiosis and helminthiasis.

Concern over Which Helminths Come to the Feed Yard with the Cattle

The importance, impact, and remediation of helminthiasis are demonstrable in all phases of the cattle industry wherein grazing is the norm, parasite transmission is ongoing, and chemical intervention is subject to assessment (FECR or control test). None of that is the case when it comes to feedlot cattle. Grazing is done, endoparasite transmission is done, and the effectiveness of anthelmintic intervention is both clouded and taken for granted. Generally, worms as a whole are not viewed as a problem at the feed yard, regardless of who they are, when they come, or where they came from. It is an eye-opening cognition to see how little respect worms receive at the feed yard. But, judging from looking at feed yard animals, helminth infections are more controlled there than at any other point in the movement of beef from the dam to the dinner table. But that is not to say that worms can be considered irrelevant at the feed yard, because they are all parasites and impart detriment to the host reflective of their speciation, stage of development, activity, and population size. Because worms are important, worm removal is likewise important, which in turn renders anthelmintic efficacy important. The remainder of this discussion is directed toward the helminths that most likely have an impact on beef production at the feed yard: their presence, impact, and efficacious removal.

Cestodes (Tapeworms)

Intestinal (strobilar) tapeworm infections are common in cattle (eg, *Moniezia benedeni*). To date, no published reports are available that document the significance of these infections. Despite this lack of documentation, it is inconceivable that strobiluses that physically cover complete sections of small intestine mucosa do not decrease FE. These cestodes are typically 2.5 m long and 1 to 2 cm wide, rarely occur singularly, and are applied to the mucosa in a fashion similar to wet wallpaper. In a survey of calves on arrival to the feed yard during the fall of 2014 (**Table 2**), more than 17% of the calves had patent infections of *M benedeni*. In a study conducted 10 years ago at the University of Arkansas (Yazwinski T.A. and Tucker C, personal communication, 2014), the authors necropsied stocker calves with as many as

Table 2
Coprology (fecal flotation) results on randomly sourced and sampled cattle entering feedlots in Nebraska, Oklahoma, and Texas in the fall of 2014 (n = 282)

	Egg Type		
	Strongyle	Nematodirus	Moniezia
Number with patent infections	279	45	49
Positive (%)	98.9	16.0	17.4
EPG range	0–9000	0–42	—
EPG AM	362.8	1.2	—
>100 EPG (%)	51.8	—	—

Abbreviation: AM, arithmetical mean.

60 scolexes, 25% of which had complete strobiluses. Regardless the significance of *M benedeni* infections at the feed yard, nothing can be done about it, because there is no cestodicide cleared for use in cattle in North America. High dose rates of benzimidazoles would be efficacious, but the levels would far surpass any realistic rates of administration.

Infections of cattle by *Cysticercus bovis* (metacestode stage of *Taenia saginata*) have been detected at abattoirs in the United States and Canada in previous years, resultant of contamination from sewer plants[6] or via fecal-oral, human contamination of cattle.[7] As is the case with strobilar infections, there is nothing that can realistically be done with cattle to clear the metacestode infections (cysticerci/bladder worms). The end results of confirmed metacestode infections are carcass condemnations at the slaughter plant and health agency inspections back along the animal supply chain.

Trematodes (Liver [and Deer] Flukes)

In most respects, the futility of anthelmintic intervention at the feed yard relative to liver fluke infection is the same as with cestode infections (ie, too late to do anything that would translate into improved feed yard economics). In a 1989 feed yard study,[8] treatment of fluke-infected animals with clorsulon at 7 mg/kg body weight (BW) (Curatrem, Merck & Co, Kenilworth, NJ) was shown to increase animal performance at the yard as well as slightly diminish the rate of liver condemnations at the packing plant. A formulation of clorsulon is not available today that delivers the drug at that dose rate. Currently, clorsulon is available only in plus formulations (combined with MLs) and is supplied at the dose rate of 2 mg/kg BW. This lower dose is not effective against juvenile *Fasciola hepatica*. Reflective of the solely adulticidal activity of clorsulon as delivered today, treatment of feed yard cattle known to have liver flukes does not result in either increased animal performance or reduced liver condemnations.[9] In the 2 clorsulon studies (cited previously), liver condemnation rates in control groups approached 80%, but it seems that the normal rate of fluke-induced liver condemnations across all carcasses is approximately 2%, with highs of 9.6% in mix-sourced cattle coming to the feed yard immediately after peak infection periods.[10,11] These peak periods of fluke transmission are during the late summer and autumn in the northwest United States[12] and during the spring to early summer in the southeast United Stsates.[13]

In addition to clorsulon, albendazole (Valbazen, Zoetis, Kalamazoo, MI), delivered at the normal dose rate of 10 mg/kg BW, has been shown effective against adult stages of *F hepatica* as well as adult stages of *Fascioloides magna*.[14] *Fascioloides magna* (the deer fluke) is common in certain sections of the United States that are generally conducive to liver fluke epidemiology but additionally augmented by healthy deer populations that share the cattle pastures.[15] Evidently, *Fascioloides magna* is not of the prevalence in the United States that approaches that of *F hepatica*, because the latter accounts for the vast majority of published reports and investigations. That said, deer fluke infections of cattle can be more prevalent that those by the liver fluke and, in some regions, account for the total fluke presence in cattle (Stromberg, personal communication, 2009).

Nematodes (Roundworms)

A vast number of nematode parasites infect cattle in North America. A select few that are most abundant are listed in **Table 1**. This discussion is weighted toward the ones in **Table 1** deemed highly likely to have an impact on animal performance and economics at the feed yard: *Cooperia punctata*, *Ostertagia ostertagi*, *Haemonchus placei*, and *Oesophagostomum radiatum*. The assessment that these particular nematodes should be the focus of this discussion is based on the authors' years of stocker calf, replacement heifer, cow-calf, and feed yard work coupled with recent coprology performed on fecal samples representative of several thousand animals received at feed yards in Oklahoma, Texas, and Nebraska during the fall of 2014 (**Fig. 1**; see **Table 2**). Of the 282 samples submitted, 98.9% contained strongyle eggs and 16.0% contained *Nematodirus helvetianus* eggs. The magnitude of *N helvetianus* egg counts were not considered high. This coupled with the fact that *Nematodirus* is limited to younger animals[16] leads the authors to believe that the thread-necked worm is of little consequence at the feed yard. Levels of strongyle eggs, however, were high, with a mean eggs per gram of feces (EPG) count of 362.8, an EPG range of 0 to 9000, and with 51.8% of the samples with an EPG greater than 100. Even though there is no absolute correlation between EPG levels and the extent of corresponding pathogenesis, the levels of nematode eggs found in the submitted samples clearly indicate that robust populations of nematode parasites routinely accompany their hosts to the feed yard (see **Fig. 1**).

For each fecal sample with an EPG count of 30 or greater, and for which sample there was a sufficient amount of feces (>30 g), a coproculture was constructed and harvested 14 days later. Results of those coproculture harvests and L3 identifications are presented in **Fig. 1**. Incidences for the strongyle species were *C punctata* greater than *O ostertagi* greater than *C oncophora* greater than *H placei* greater than *Oesophagostomum radiatum*. Across all harvests, 49.1% of the L3 were *C punctata*, 18.2% *H placei*, 15.5% *C oncophora*, 14.8% *O ostertagi*, and 2.8% *O radiatum*. *Trichostrongylus axei* was of minor profile in regard to incidence or abundance.

The nematodes of considerable presence, as discussed previously, are the same ones found in stocker calf systems, an obvious parallel because cattle get loaded onto the trailers at the stocker/backgrounder operations as stocker calves and are delivered to the feed yards a day later as feed yard cattle. The perceived significance of these nematodes, however, is greatly diminished with that truck ride. These worms, however, have considerable impact at the feed yard, with species-specific considerations.

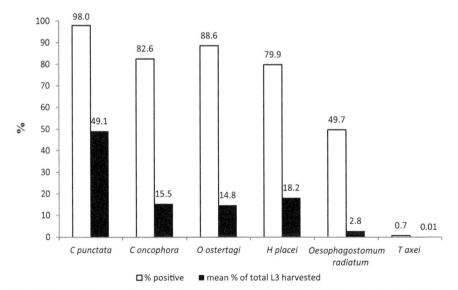

Fig. 1. Coproculture results on randomly sourced and sampled cattle entering feedlots in Nebraska, Oklahoma, and Texas in the fall of 2014 (149 individual animal coprocultures made from 282 individual animal fecal samples).

Judging from the coprology data, discussed previously, the *Cooperia* spp (*C oncophora* and *C punctata*) are both of high incidence and fecundity in cattle received at the feed yard. Both are extremely capable pathogens.[17,18] Additionally, the *Cooperia* spp have the distinction of being the cattle nematodes most often documented as resistant to the MLs.[19] In the early 1980s in Arkansas, *C oncophora* was the predominant *Cooperia* sp in stocker cattle. At the turn of the century, *C punctata* became the most abundant of the genus. Given the likelihood that *C oncophora* and/or *C punctata* are in the cattle as they enter the feed yard, and that these nematodes also most likely are ML resistant, the use of a benzimidazole (fenbendazole, oxfendazole, or albendazole) or an imidazothiazole (levamisole) at receiving, in addition to an ML, is indicated. Three additional observations should be made regarding the *Cooperia* spp in cattle. First, they are fairly restricted to younger animals.[20,21] By the time animals get to the feed yard, their *Cooperia* spp infections are low compared with earlier infections or are declining without any chemical intervention. Second, even though the *Cooperia* most likely are ML resistant, the resistance is more focused against the avermectins than against moxidectin.[22] These investigators state, "resistance to avermectins and to moxidectin is becoming common in *Cooperia* spp, especially *C oncophora* in cattle around the world, although moxidectin remains more effective than avermectins once resistance is detected." Lastly, there is evidence that ML-resistant *Cooperia* spp are more pathogenic than their ML-sensitive counterparts.[23,24] Given the ubiquity of *Cooperia* spp infections in incoming cattle and this last observation concerning the connection between pathogenicity and resistance, *Cooperia* spp infections should be one of the targets of a receiving anthelmintic regime.

O ostertagi is another nematode listed as highly likely to have an impact on animal performance at the feed yard. At the turn of the century, the impression in Arkansas was that *O ostertagi* burdens were on the decline, an observation shared by many in North America. These impressions sadly have proved erroneous. Recent work in arkansas,[25] observations by others, detection of ML resistance by *O ostertagi* in the northwest,[26] and the coprology results discussed previously all clearly indicate that the brown stomach worm should continue to be considered in any scheme of anthelmintic intervention regardless of animal age or husbandry. In addition, the type of ostertagiasis must be considered when it comes to animal treatment at the feed yard,[27,28] with pronounced, seasonal inhibition following northern or southern trends and with only the MLs effective against inhibited stages when treatment is given at normal, label-inscribed dose rates.[29] Given the normal tenure of cattle at the feed yard (approximately 150 days), populations of inhibited *O ostertagi*, which are not removed by the receiving treatment(s), most likely have sufficient time before slaughter to resume development and instigate type 2 ostertagiasis, the most debilitative form of ostertagiasis.[30,31]

H placei seems the primary barber pole worm of cattle in North America.[32] Over the past 3 decades, *Haemonchus* spp infections in North American cattle have definitely progressed in 2 regards: (1) the endemic zone has expanded from the south (primarily Texas) to Wisconsin and all points in between and (2), the genus has become resistant to both benzimidazoles and the MLs.[33] Their state of anthelmintic resistance in receiving cattle at the feed yard is equal to or greater than that shown by the *Cooperia* spp.[34] As with the *Cooperia* spp, effective elimination of *H placei* at the feed yard is probably best accomplished by treatment with a combination of benzimidazole (or imidazothiazole) with an ML. Even though *H placei* burdens have been extended across a majority of the United States, it is likely that their severity is diminished the more north the grazing is conducted.

The final nematode that is listed as most likely to have an impact on cattle at the feed yard is *Oesophagostomum radiatum* (the nodular worm). Little mention in the literature has been made concerning this nematode in recent years. Judging from the numerous coprology and necropsy studies the authors have done over the years, this nematode is estimated to have approximately 80% prevalence in Arkansas. Additionally, the authors have found nodular worm infections to persist even after repeated benzimidazole treatments (unpublished observations). *Oesophagostomum* spp L3 can infect transcutaneous (a route also used by infective larvae of cattle hookworms and threadworms) and has been cited as a nematode that can persist and infect under feedlot conditions.[35] Actual documentation of the feed yard cycling of nodular worm infections, or the cycling of any nematode at feed yard, has not been published.

Anthelmintics in Use at the Feed Yard

Judging from the answers received from the questionnaire, and in consideration of the nematodes to target for treatment at receiving (discussed previously), the most fail-safe receiving anthelmintic regime is a combination of benzimidazole (or imidazothiazole) and ML. The benzimidazole or imidazothiazole serves to remove the nematodes resistant to the MLs, the MLs remove the arrested nematodes and help control the lice, and the combinational effects are directed against the rest of the nematodes. Regardless of what is given at receiving (ML, benzimidazole, imidazothiazole, pioneer, or generic) the overwhelming conclusion drawn from the questionnaire answers is that "worms are not a problem from the point of receiving on." Unfortunately, there are significant differences in efficacy between the nematocides as used in cattle.[29] In turn, these differences in drug efficacy translate into differing levels of nematodes infecting the cattle for the duration of time spent at the feed yard. Because the ill effects of worms at the feed yard have not routinely been observed, it seems that the lion's share of the pathologic effects of nematode parasites at the feed yard (left behind due to the use of nonefficacious anthelmintics) are greatly diminished as an indirect effect of enhanced animal resilience (tissue repair and replacement) and resistance (immunity and inflammation); this is due to the high quality and quantity of the feed (protein, energy, and so forth) given at the feed yard. The effect of improved nutrition reducing the deleterious effects of gastrointestinal (GI) parasitisms has been known for some time.[36] Additionally, at the feed yard, there might be something more—a direct effect of unnatural diet and chyme that are abruptly placed on the nematodes. The capstone event of immunologically driven nematode expulsion is the "weep and sweep", wherein the environment of the nematode becomes too averse for the nematodes to maintain position. There must be an abrupt change in the physical nature of chyme experienced by the GI nematodes as the stocker calf (pasture-based diet) becomes housed at the feed yard (concentrate-based diet). An illustration of this exact scenario was obtained with a set of calves followed from receiving to harvest.[34] No statistically significant efficacy was in evidence for a generic ivermectin given at receiving. Yet all fecal nematode egg counts dropped by 90%, and the animals performed within acceptable norms for ADG, FE, and carcass traits. Additionally, when a subset of treated animals was put back on a hay diet, their egg counts returned to pretreatment/prefeedlot levels. Something is definitely happening at the feed yard wherein the adverse effects of nematodes are diluted. Truly, the need is there for more research provided the interest, funding, and willingness to include appropriate control groups can be found. Parasites, let behind by ineffective anthelmintics, do not cease being parasites at the feed yard. Their presence, measured at some level, must be directly related to a reduction of calf performance.

The direct, negative correlation between worms at the feed yard and the performance of cattle at the feed yard was obtained in a 1997 study conducted in Oklahoma and Texas.[37,38] Control and treated groups of stocker calves were followed for a 118-day grazing period. Immediately after grazing, the cattle were delivered to feedlot and subdivided within prior treatment group to control and treatment groups again, after which time they were followed for 121 days at the feed yard prior to harvest (and quantification of abomasum nematodes). Ultimately, therefore, 4 different treatment groups of calves were achieved: (1) not treated at pasture or feedlot, (2) treated only at feedlot, (3) treated only at pasture, and (4) treated both at pasture and feedlot. The data from this study are presented in **Figs. 2** and **3**. For both the size of nematode populations at harvest and percent of animals pulled for miscellaneous treatments during feed yard (primarily respiratory), the groups were 1 greater than 2 greater than 3 greater than 4 (see **Fig. 2**). The more nematodes in the calves during feed yard, the more the calves were prone to develop secondary disease. Production parameters (ADG, FE, and dry matter intake [DMI]; see **Fig. 3**) could also be directly sorted to nematode levels but with the influence of what seems to have been a compensatory effect as well. For both grazing groups (dewormed vs controls), treatment at feedlot improved animal performance, but the improvement was most pronounced when wormy calves were treated as opposed to when clean calves were treated. ADG, FE, and DMI were improved by feedlot treatments of untreated pasture calves by 13.4%, 4.9%, and 7.1%, respectively. Corresponding improvements seen for feedlot treatment of pasture-treated calves were 4.2%, 0.3%, and 2.8%,

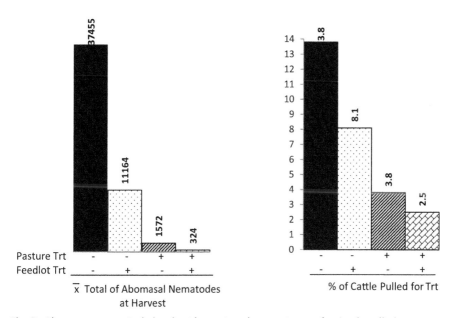

$\overline{x}$ Total of Abomasal Nematodes
at Harvest

% of Cattle Pulled for Trt

Fig. 2. Abomasum nematode levels at harvest and percentages of animals pulled per treatment group for health anomalies during feedlot. Trt, treatment. (*Data from* Smith RA, Rogers KC, Huse S, et al. Pasture deworming and (or) subsequent feedlot deworming with fenbendazole. I. Effects on grazing performance, feedlot performance and carcass traits of yearling steers. Bov Pract 2000;34:104–14; and Taylor RF, Bliss DH, Brandt RT, et al. Pasture deworming and (or) subsequent feedlot deworming with fenbendazole. II. Effects on abomasal worm counts and abomasal pathology of yearling steers. Bov Pract 2000;34:115–23.)

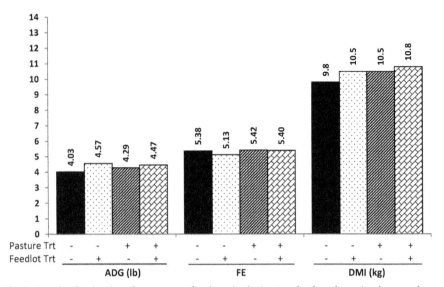

Fig. 3. Levels of animal performance at feed yard relative to whether the animals were dewormed on pasture before feed yard, at reception to the feed yard, or both. (*Data from* Smith RA, Rogers KC, Huse S, et al. Pasture deworming and (or) subsequent feedlot deworming with fenbendazole. I. Effects on grazing performance, feedlot performance and carcass traits of yearling steers. Bov Pract 2000;34:104–14.)

respectively. The ill effects of worms and the impact of compensatory responsiveness (a much used trait by most if not all cattle buyers) were illustrated in this study (see **Figs. 2** and **3**).

Finally, regarding anthelmintics, is the topic of assessing anthelmintic effectiveness at the feedlot. Anthelmintic efficacies are generally determined via the FECR test or the control test. The control test is the test of choice, because the actual parasite burdens in the control and treated group(s) are quantified at necropsy and used to directly determine drug efficacy. Due to costing, this test is rarely done, especially at the feed yard. The FECR test, therefore, is the most acceptable test, but, as discussed previously, the abrupt change of animal diet coincident with anthelmintic treatment at the feed yard would most likely cloud the assessment of drug effectiveness, especially if a control group was not used.

Pertaining to fecal egg counts at the feed yard, and in a broader sense to the overall concern at the feed yard regarding worms, during a recent round table of consulting veterinarians convened in Kansas, the documentation and assessment of GI parasitisms was discussed and the pros and cons of fecal egg counts debated. At the end of the round table, one of the veterinarians stated, "it's been over 20 years since I've done an egg count." By itself, that statement attests to the concern people at the feed yard have regarding worms, a testament to the subclinical nature of the disease and how its impact is hidden, even in a production system that is monitored and regulated to the nth degree for optimal animal health and productivity.

SUMMARY

Fly and louse infestations are readily discerned and remedied in feedlot cattle. Tapeworm and fluke infections are accepted as probable, but, given the lack of anthelmintics with realistic efficacy against these infections, these helminths are allowed to persist without treatment. Nematode infections are considered ubiquitous with cattle coming from pasture and are targeted with an ML, usually in combination with a benzimidazole. Not identified in the receiving cattle are populations of ML-resistant worms, benzimidazole-resistant worms, and worms in arrestment. Regardless, these subpopulations of nematodes seem effectively controlled by a combination of anthelmintic treatment, animal resistance and resilience, lack of reinfection, and diet. The bottom line is that a great job of parasite control is being conducted by the feedlot industry. More needs to be done, however, at the feed yard as well as for the feed yard, such as (1) the development of a new flukicide that targets immature and mature stages, (2) the development of a cestocide that targets strobilar infections, (3) the quantification of nematode burdens (arrested, resistant, susceptible, and so forth) with corresponding nematocidal efficaces, and (4), the development of a combination product (benzimidazole/imidazothiazole plus ML) that can be given as one application.

ACKNOWLEDGMENTS

Linda Jones, an Administrative Specialist at University of Arkansas, made substantial contributions to this article.

REFERENCES

1. Peel DS. Beef cattle growing and backgrounding programs. Vet Clin North Am Food Anim Pract 2003;19:365–85.
2. Greene GL, Sloderbeck PE, Nechols JR. Biological fly control for Kansas feedlots. MF 2223. Manhattan, NY: Kansas State University Cooperative Extension Service; 1998. Available at: http://www.oznet.ksu.edu.
3. Floate KD, Fox AS. Indirect effects of ivermectin residues across trophic levels. Musca domestica (Diptera: Muscidae) and Muscidifurax zaraptor (Hymenoptera: Pteromalidae). Bull Entomol Res 1999;89:225–9.
4. Ernst JV, Benz GW. Intestinal coccidiosis in cattle. Vet Clin North Am Food Anim Pract 1986;2:283–91.
5. Lucas AS, Swecker WS, Lindsay DS, et al. A study of the level and dynamics of Eimeria populations in naturally infected, grazing beef cattle at various stages of production in the Mid-Atlantic USA. Vet Parasitol 2014;202:201–6.
6. Lees W, Nightingale J, Brown D, et al. Outbreak of Cysticercus bovis (Taenia saginata) in feedlot cattle in Alberta. Can Vet J 2002;43:227–8.
7. Hoberg EP. Taenia tapeworms: their biology, evolution and socioeconomic significance. Microbes Infect 2002;4:859–66.
8. Johnson EG. Effects of liver flukes on feedlot performance. Agri Pract 1991;12: 33–6.
9. Johnson EG, Rowland WK, Zimmerman GL, et al. Performance of feedlot cattle with parasite burdens treated with anthelmintics. Comp Cont Educ Pract Vet 1998;20:116–23.
10. Brown TR, Laurence TE. Association of liver abnormalities with carcass grading performance and value. J Anim Sci 2010;88:4037–43.
11. McKeith RO, Gray GD, Hale DS, et al. National beef quality audit – 2011; harvest-floor assessments of targeted characteristics that affect quality and value of cattle, carcasses, and byproducts. J Anim Sci 2012;90:5135–42.
12. Hoover RC, Lincoln SD, Hall RF, et al. Seasonal transmission of Fasciola hepatica to cattle in northwestern United States. J Am Vet Med Assoc 1984; 184:695–8.

13. Malone JB, Loyacano AF, Hugh-Jones ME, et al. A three-year study on seasonal transmission and control of Fasciola hepatica of cattle in Louisiana. Prev Vet Med 1984;3:131–41.
14. Craig TM, Qureshi T, Miller DK, et al. Efficacy of two formulations of albendazole against liver flukes in cattle. Am J Vet Res 1992;53:1170–1.
15. Craig TM, Bell RR. Seasonal transmission of liver flukes to cattle in the Texas gulf coast. J Am Vet Med Assoc 1978;173:104–7.
16. Herlich H. Age resistance of cattle to nematodes of the gastrointestinal tract. J Parasitol 1960;46:392–7.
17. Armour J, Bairden K, Homes PH, et al. Pathophysiological and parasitological studies on Cooperia oncophora infections in calves. Res Vet Sci 1987;42:373–81.
18. Sromberg BE, Gasbarre LC, Waite A, et al. Cooperia punctata: effect on cattle productivity? Vet Parasitol 2012;183:284–91.
19. Kaplan RM, Vidyashankar AN. An inconvenient truth: global worming and anthelmintic resistance. Vet Parasitol 2012;186:70–8.
20. Roberts FH, O'Sullivan PJ, Riek RF. The epidemiology of parasitic gastroenteritis of cattle. Aust J Agric Res 1952;3:187–225.
21. Claerebout E, Dorny P, Agneesens J, et al. The effect of first season chemoprophylaxis in calves on second season pasture contamination and acquired resistance and resilience to gastrointestinal nematodes. Vet Parasitol 1999;80:289–301.
22. Prichard R, Menez C, Lespine A. Moxidectin and the avermectins: consanguinity but not identity. Int J Parasitol 2012;2:134–53.
23. Coles GC, Watson CL, Anziani OS. Ivermectin-resistant Cooperia in cattle. Vet Rec 2001;148:283–4.
24. Njue AI, Prichard RK. Efficacy of ivermectin in calves against a resistant Cooperia oncophora field isolate. Parasitol Res 2004;93:419–22.
25. Yazwinski TA, Beck P, Tucker C, et al. Treatment of stocker calves at turnout with an eprinomectin extended-release injection or a combination of injectable doramectin and oral albendazole. AAVP Proc Abst No 33. Denver, July 26-29, 2014.
26. Edmonds MD, Johnson EG, Edmonds JD. Anthelmintic resistance of Ostertagia ostertagi and Cooperia oncophora to macrocyclic lactones in cattle from the western United States. Vet Parasitol 2010;170:224–9.
27. Gibbs HC. The epidemiology of bovine Ostertagiasis in the north temperate regions of North American. Vet Parasitol 1988;27:39–47.
28. Williams JC, Knox JW, Baumann BA, et al. Seasonal changes of gastrointestinal nematode populations in yearling beef cattle in Louisiana with emphasis on prevalence of inhibition in Ostertagia ostertagi. Int J Parasitol 1983;13:133–43.
29. Yazwinski TA, Tucker CA, Powell J, et al. Fecal egg count reduction and control trial determinations of anthelmintic efficacies for several parasiticides utilizing a single set of naturally infected calves. Vet Parasitol 2009;164:232–41.
30. Anderson N, Armour J, Jarrett WF, et al. Experimental infections of Ostertagia ostertagi in calves: results of two regimes of multiple inoculations. Am J Vet Res 1967;28:1073–7.
31. Armour J, Jennings FW, Urquhart GM. Inhibition of Ostertagia ostertagi at the early fourth stage I. The seasonal incidence. Res Vet Sci 1969;10:232–7.
32. Chaudhry U, Miller M, Yazwinski T, et al. The presence of benzimidazole resistance mutations in Haemonchus placei from US cattle. Vet Parasitol 2014;204:411–5.
33. Yazwinski TA, Tucker CA. A sampling of factors relative to the epidemiology of gastrointestinal nematode parasites of cattle in the United States. Vet Clin North Am Food Anim Pract 2006;22:501–27.

34. Yazwinski TA, Tucker CA, Miles DG, et al. Evaluation of generic injectable ivermectin for control of nematodiasis in feedlot heifers. Bov Pract 2012;46:60–5.
35. Gasharre LC. Anthelmintic resistance in cattle nematodes in the US. Vet Parasitol 2014;204:3–11.
36. Goldberg A. The relationship of diet to GI helminth parasitism in cattle. Am J Vet Res 1959;20:806–14.
37. Smith RA, Rogers KC, Huse S, et al. Pasture deworming and (or) subsequent feedlot deworming with fenbendazole. I. Effects on grazing performance, feedlot performance and carcass traits of yearling steers. Bov Pract 2000;34:104–14.
38. Taylor RF, Bliss DH, Brandt RT, et al. Pasture deworming and (or) subsequent feedlot deworming with fenbendazole. II. Effects on abomasal worm counts and abomasal pathology of yearling steers. Bov Pract 2000;34:115–23.

Management of Cattle Exposed to Adverse Environmental Conditions

Terry L. Mader, MS, PhD[a],*, Dee Griffin, DVM, MS[a,b]

KEYWORDS

- Environmental stress • Animal welfare • Livestock management

KEY POINTS

- Domestic livestock that are traditionally managed outdoors are particularly vulnerable not only to extreme environmental conditions but also to rapid changes in these conditions.
- Management and facility alternatives need to be considered to help these animals cope with adverse conditions.
- Manipulation of dietary ingredients, energy density, and intake may also be beneficial for livestock challenged by environmental conditions.
- Under hot conditions, high-volume water-holding devices and water availability is of upmost importance.
- Under cold conditions, maintaining facilities that prevent animals from getting wet/muddy is of upmost importance.

INTRODUCTION

Ruminants have the ability to generate a substantial amount of heat through fermentation of feedstuffs. In particular, high-producing animals fed high-energy diets generate large amounts of metabolic heat, which is usually transferred from the body to the environment using normal physiologic processes. Failure to transfer this heat in the summer results in an accumulation of heat within the body and predisposes the animal to heat stress.[1,2] This stress can cause animal discomfort or even death in the summer, whereas preservation of body heat results in an opposite effect in the winter. Regardless of season, under extreme environmental conditions, management of livestock discomfort and potential for deaths must be a higher priority than performance losses. Animal discomfort and related heat flux management can be achieved

The Authors have nothing to disclose.
[a] University of Nebraska-Lincoln, Lincoln, NE 68028, USA; [b] Great Plains Veterinary Educational Center, Clay Center, NE 68933, USA
* Corresponding author. 9301 Valaretta Drive, Gretna, NE 68028, USA.
E-mail address: tmader1@unl.edu

through behavioral changes initiated by the animal or facilities and/or feed management changes initiated by the caretaker.[3–5]

The primary objective of any environmental mitigation strategy is to aid the animal in the winter to keep the body temperature (BT) elevated throughout the day and in the summer to reduce the peak BT during the day and/or help the animal drive the BT down at night (**Fig. 1**). Studies, reported herein, were conducted under harsh environmental conditions, either in laboratory or natural environments, in an effort to better understand animal responses to those conditions and develop mitigation strategies for those conditions.

GENERAL GUIDELINES
Pen Layout

Proper feedlot pen layout and design are crucial for minimizing the effects of adverse climates. Mounds need to be built into feedlot pens, especially in the northern plains and western Corn Belt of the United States to minimize mud problems during wet periods and enhance airflow during hot periods. In the southern plains, mounds are not as crucial to have in feedlot pens; nevertheless, to enhance drainage and minimize buildup of mud and other residue, a slope of 3% to 4% away from the bunks is recommended. Also, proper design and strategic use of windbreaks is warranted.[6] Wind barriers or other structures should not be placed near (~30 m from pen) cattle in the summer in order to maximize airflow in the pen and around the animal.

Stocking Density for Mud and Dust Control

Even though mud tends to be a winter/spring problem and dust a summer/fall problem, both can be problematic year-round in some areas of the country. The degree to which

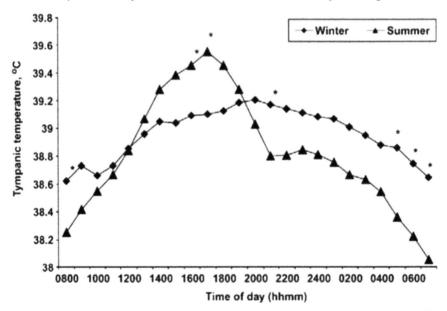

Fig. 1. Effects of season on tympanic temperature over a 24-hour period in feedlot heifers. Asterisks indicate that means within an hour differ by season ($P<.05$; SE = 0.10). Each point represents the mean of 12 pens of cattle. (*Data from* Mader TL, Kreikemeier WM. Effects of growth-promoting agents and season on blood metabolites and body temperature in heifers. J Anim Sci 2006;84:1030–7.)

these occur depends on the level or amount of moisture in the feedlot soil surface. Dust will tend to be a greater problem in areas where evaporation exceeds precipitation, whereas mud will be a greater problem where precipitation exceeds evaporation. Dust is relatively easy to control through sprinkling of the feedlot surface or by increasing cattle density in the pen through cross-fencing or shortening the pen. Decreasing pen space allows more urine/water to be deposited per unit of space, thus mitigating dust through adhesion and preventing fine particles from lifting off the feedlot surface.

Mud is much more difficult to control and in some months requires a much greater level of input to manage. If you target your management activities on mud control back in the summer when it is dry you will fare much better the following season when it is wet. Cleaning pens of manure (undigested residues that act like a sponge to retain water) is essential for maintaining a firm base. Filling in holes and rebuilding upper portions of the pens with a combination of clay soil and old manure is needed.

Stocking densities of around 7 m^2 (75 ft^2) are often sufficient to control dust in pens containing heavy feedlot cattle in the summer. However, for cattle fed under outside conditions, stocking densities greater than 35 m^2 (>375 ft^2) may be needed in wet areas of the country to minimize mud, but this in itself will often not eliminate it.

SUMMER MITIGATION STRATEGIES

Improved cattle welfare during periods of hot weather depends, in part, on the timely assessment of animal status in regard to heat load. Panting score (PS) has been found to be an easy and effective method for assessing heat-related animal discomfort.[3] The PS system (**Table 1**) assesses the respiratory dynamics of cattle using a 4 point system 0, 1, 2, 3, 4.[3,7]

Studies have used PS to assess heat load in feedlot cattle and have shown a direct relationship between environmental thermal load and PS.[3,8] In addition, Brown-Brandl and colleagues[9] and Gaughan and colleagues[1] reported that PS was a good visual

Table 1
PS and panting score descriptor

PS	Descriptor
0 (No stress)	No panting
1 (Mild stress)	Slight panting, mouth closed, no drool, easy to see chest movements
2 (Moderate stress)	Fast panting, drool present (from nose and mouth), no open mouth, easy to see chest movements
2.5 (Moderate stress)	As for 2, but occasional open mouth, tongue not extended
3 (Severe stress)	Open mouth and excessive drooling, neck extended, head held up, tongue not extended, rapid panting rate
3.5 (Severe stress)	As for 3, but with tongue out slightly and occasionally fully extended for short periods
4 (Extreme stress)	Open mouth with tongue fully extended for prolonged periods, excessive drooling, neck extended and head held up, may shift to deeper breathing with reduction in panting rate for short periods
4.5 (Catastrophic stress)	As for 4, head often lowered, shift to deeper breathing, cattle struggling to breath, panting rate slows, drooling may cease

Adapted from Mader TL, Davis MS, Brown-Brandl T. Environmental factors influencing heat stress in feedlot cattle. J Anim Sci 2006;84:712–9; and Gaughan JB, Mader TL, Holt SM, et al. A new heat load index for feedlot cattle. J Anim Sci 2008;86:226–34.

method for determining differences in thermal tolerance between cattle breeds. In addition, Gaughan and Mader[10] found a strong relationship between PS and BT (Equation 1):

$$y = 39.01 + 0.38x \ (R^2 = 0.68; \ P<.001) \tag{1}$$

where y = BT (°C) and x = PS.

A quadratic relationship was found between BT and PS when considered by the time-of-day category (morning [AM], midday [MD], or afternoon [PM]) (Equations 2–4). These relationships are presented in the following equations, and the relationship between BT and PS is shown graphically in **Fig. 2.**

$$(AM): y = 39.08 + 0.009x + 0.137x^2 \ (R^2 = 0.94; \ P<.001) \tag{2}$$

$$(MD): y = 39.09 + 0.914x - 0.080x^2 \ (R^2 = 0.89; \ P<.001) \tag{3}$$

$$(PM): y = 39.52 + 0.790x - 0.068x^2 \ (R^2 = 0.83; \ P<.001) \tag{4}$$

The strong correlation between BT and PS in the current study confirms that PS is a good management tool for the assessment of heat load in cattle. Furthermore, relationships among BT, PS, and respiration rate have been defined further to provide producers with additional information in assessing animal discomfort as a tool in heat-stress mitigation management.[10,11] Substantial details on the improvement in and development of new environmental stress indices, which are related to various environmental conditions and/or PS, have been published by Eigenberg and colleagues,[12] Mader and colleagues,[2,3] and Gaughan and colleagues.[7]

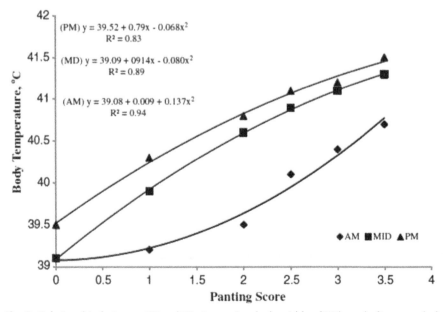

Fig. 2. Relationship between BT and PS at morning (AM), midday (MD), and afternoon (PM): entire study. (*Adapted from* Gaughan JB, Mader TL. Body temperature and respiratory dynamics in un-shaded beef cattle. Int J Biometeor 2014;58(7):1448; with permission.)

Restricted or Managed Feeding Programs

Benefits of using restricted feeding programs under hot conditions have been reported by Mader and colleagues[13] and Davis and colleagues.[14] In addition, Reinhardt and Brandt[15] found the use of restricted feeding programs to be particularly effective when cattle were fed late afternoon or evening versus morning. Implementing a bunk management regimen, whereby bunks are kept empty 4 to 6 hours during the daytime hours is another management strategy that could be used to minimize peak metabolic heat load occurring simultaneously to peak climatic heat load.[16] Even though this forces the cattle to eat in the evening, it does not seem to increase nighttime BT. In restricted feeding studies in which BT was measured, Mader and colleagues[17] housed feedlot steers under thermoneutral or hot environmental conditions. Steers were offered a 6%-roughage finishing diet ad libitum (HE), offered the same diet restricted at 85% to 90% of ad libitum dry matter intake (DMI) levels (RE), or offered a 28%-roughage diet ad libitum (HR). Steers fed the HR diet (39.7°C/103.5°F) had significantly lower BT under hot conditions than HE-fed (40.6°C/105.1°F) and RE-fed (40.3°C/104.5°F) steers, whereas RE-fed steers had significantly lower BT than HE-fed steers. The lower BT of the HR- and RE-fed steers would indicate that metabolizable energy intake before exposure to excessive heat load influences the ability of cattle to cope with the challenge of hot environments and that lowering ME intake can lower BT.[14] Arias and colleagues[18] reported similar results in that high-concentrate feedlot diets (3.04 megacalories ME/kg) promoted greater BT in the summer, whereas the lower-energy higher-roughage diets (2.63 megacalories ME/kg) tended to produce lower BT in the winter.

Heat-Increment Management

Heat production increases with digestion and metabolism, which is known as *heat increment*. Heat increment can be thought of as energy that must be dissipated. Dissipating this heat is not really a problem under thermoneutral or cold environmental conditions. However, under high heat load, in which the animal's ability to dissipate body heat is impaired, additional body heat may be detrimental to the animal's well-being. Feed ingredients differ in heat increment, largely because of differences in the efficiency of utilization of the nutrient or the end products of digestion. For example, fibrous feedstuffs have greater heat increments (per unit of ME) than feedstuffs containing more soluble carbohydrates. In theory, it is possible to formulate diets according to heat increment; but evidence on whether this practice is effective in alleviating heat stress in feedlot cattle is inconclusive. The previous discussion would suggest that in total the amount of heat generated from feeding a lower-energy moderate-fiber diet is less than that generated from a high-concentrate diet. The addition of dietary fat would seem to be the best alternative for reducing heat increment because fat has a low heat increment. In beef cattle studies, mixed results have been found for steers exposed to high heat load and fed grain diets high in fat.[19]

Water Temperature Concerns

Under mob and cell grazing situations, aboveground water lines and small, dark-colored water-holding vessels can significantly increase water temperature and water requirements. An experiment carried out at the University of New England (Armidale, New South Wales, Australia) with Merino wethers found that drinking-water temperature can affect water intake.[20] Analyses of water preference data revealed that in hot conditions, sheep drank considerably more ($P<.05$) 30°C water (6708 g/d) than 20°C water (1185 g/d). In the cool conditions, water intake was numerically greater ($P<.095$) from the 20°C water (4024 g/d) than from the 30°C water (2646 g/d). This study indicates that under hot conditions a greater quantity of water is required to cool animals as water temperature increases. Producers need to be sensitive to the effects of water temperature in storage devices and ensure that adequate waterer capacity and space is available for animals. Smaller water containers tend to limit water access and availability.

Waterer Space Requirements

Evaporation of moisture from the skin surface (sweating) or respiratory tract (panting) is the primary mechanism used by the animal to lose excess body heat in a hot environment.[10] Under these conditions, waterer space availability and water intake per head becomes very important. During heat episodes, Mader and colleagues[21] found that as much as 3 times the normal waterer space (7.5 cm [3.0 in] vs 2.5 cm [1.0 in] of linear space per animal) may be needed to allow for sufficient room for all animals to access and benefit from available water. In general, water consumption per unit of DMI in the summer is 2 times greater than in the winter.

Sprinkling Systems

In addition to pen design and altering feeding regimen, sprinkling can also be effective in minimizing heat stress. Benefits of sprinkling tend to be enhanced if sprinkling is started in the morning, before cattle get hot.[14] These data also show significant benefits to sprinkling or wetting pen surfaces. Sprinkling of pen surfaces may be more beneficial than sprinkling the cattle. Kelly and colleagues[22] reported feedlot ground surface temperatures in excess of 65°C by 1400 hours in the afternoon in Southern California. Similar surface temperatures can be found in most High Plains feedlots under dry conditions with high solar radiation levels. Cooling the surface would seem to provide a heat sink for cattle to dissipate body heat, thus allowing cattle to better adapt to environmental conditions versus adapting to being wetted. Wetting or sprinkling cattle can have adverse effects, particularly when the cattle get acclimated to being wet and failed or incomplete sprinkling occurs during subsequent hot days. Elevated relative humidity may also be problematic if large areas of the feedlot are sprinkled versus isolated areas in pens.

Sprinkling may increase feedlot water usage 2 to 3 fold.[23] In addition, mud buildup is associated with sprinkling systems. Intermittent sprinkling is recommended and constitutes a 2- to 5-minute application every 30 to 45 minutes or up to a 20-minute application every hour to 1.5 hours. Whether cattle that need to be sprinkled (cooled) always go to or get under the sprinklers is unknown.

Use of Shade

Shade has also been found to be beneficial for feedlot cattle exposed to hot climatic conditions.[24] In general, the response to shade is greatest at the onset of heat stress even though shade use increases with the time cattle are on feed. This finding indicates that cattle must adapt to shade or social order around and under shade before optimum shade use occurs. Although no heat-related cattle deaths occurred in this study, these results indicate that shade improves performance in the summer particularly when cattle are fed in facilities that restrict airflow and for cattle that have not become, or had the opportunity to become, acclimated to hot conditions. Sullivan and colleagues[25] found that access to shade improved the welfare and performance of the cattle. However, provision of a shade area greater than 2.0 m² per animal did not seem to provide any additional production benefits for short-fed cattle. Nevertheless, the PS and behavioral data, especially during the heat waves, indicate that the 2.0 m² per animal treatment did not produce the same welfare improvements as the 3.3 and 4.7 m^2 per animal treatments.

Greater benefits of using shade are found in areas having greater temperature and/ or solar radiation.[26] Mitlöhner and colleagues[27] found excellent results to providing shade for cattle fed near Lubbock, Texas. The overall economic benefit of using shade depends not only on location but also on the cost of structures and maintenance.

Mitigation Strategy Economic Analysis

The economic effects of imposing various environmental stress mitigation strategies have been determined by Mader[28–30] based on the comprehensive climate index[2] and how the respective mitigation strategy changes the apparent or *feels like* temperature. In the summer analysis, moderate sprinkling was used versus heavy sprinkling in an effort to minimize the quantity of excess runoff water. The pen area sprinkled was kept to around 2.3 m^2 per head. In addition to shade and sprinklers, evaluation of the use of fans (with water injection under shade) was conducted to determine the benefits of added evaporative cooling potential through the enhanced airflow under shade. From this analysis, the performance effects of sprinkling and shade on apparent temperatures were similar even though different physiologic cooling properties are involved between the two strategies. Greater amounts of water tend to have a greater benefit than shade, whereas lesser amounts (ie, misting) tend to have less benefit than shade.

Because of the limited heat tolerance of British crossbred cattle, they tended to have greater cost of gain (COG), under heat stress, than Holsteins; an opposite scenario occurs under cold stress, with Holsteins having greater COG.[29] An analysis of Brahman cross cattle displayed a lower benefit and one-time setup costs (break-even construction cost) when compared with comparable costs for other breed types.[29]

In theory, sprinkling should always produce greater heat stress relief than shade or misting because of the high heat loss associated with the evaporation process. However, limited research data in feedlot cattle indicate that shade provides a greater and more consistent performance response than sprinkling. When cattle are in very close confinement and the probability is great that water gets applied to the animal, then a more positive response to sprinkling or direct water application is found (eg, dairy units). Well-designed and constructed shade and shelters tend to produce greater long-term benefits than sprinklers and/or less stable shade structures.

Heat stress depends not only on temperature and solar radiation but also on humidity and wind speed.[31–33] Adjustments for solar radiation and wind speed have also been developed and need to be considered when predicting heat stress.[3,34] The effects of environmental stress not only depend on the magnitude and duration but also on the rate at which environmental conditions change.

COLD MITIGATION STRATEGIES

When winter conditions are severe enough, productivity is compromised as a result of increased maintenance energy requirements associated with exposure to cold, wet, and/or windy conditions. For most animals reared in the United States in outside environments, maintenance energy requirements are approximately 20% greater, respectively, in the winter than in the summer[35] (National Research Council, 2000). In addition, under winter conditions, if an animal's coat cover is wet and muddy, then energy requirements for maintenance can easily double, particularly if the animal is not protected from the wind.

Bedding and Pen Space

There are several things that can be done in the winter to enhance animal comfort. Bedding, such as crop residues or sawdust, can be used to help insulate cattle from the cold ground during severe cold outbreaks. One to 2 to 4 lb of bedding per head per day can make a big improvement in productivity. A summary of Colorado and South Dakota data found that gains and feed efficiencies can be improved nearly 7% through the use of bedding.[36] The more significant responses came during the later versus early portion of the feeding period. This finding is likely caused by problems heavier cattle often experience with wet, muddy conditions, which accompany late winter and early spring precipitation events. Lighter cattle, once they are on feed, are generally not impacted as much.

Under today's cattle feeding environment, the daily feed cost to maintain an animal that is partially wet, under winter conditions, is up to 3 times the cost of the bedding needed to keep the animal dry. Bedding is a relatively cheap alternative, especially if hay, corn, or other feed prices are relatively high when compared with bedding cost. Furthermore, once the animal is dry, bedding usage decreases, whereas if bedding is not used, the moisture-laden facilities usually remain wet and the animal stays wet. However, the benefits of bedding are diminished when ample space is provided for the cattle. In studies conducted in Nebraska, it was found that doubling normal pen space (>46 m^2/500 ft^2) in the winter was as effective as using bedding.[37] Some cattle operations do not have the luxury of doubling space, and there is not a desire to bed cattle. Nevertheless, at the very least, young animals or animals that are susceptible to getting sick are candidates for bedding. If bedding is used, the bedded areas must be cleaned periodically. In addition, livestock should be provided with as much dry area as possible to allow them to spread out and lay down. The more concentrated the animals are under wet conditions, the less chance there will be for surfaces to dry, which will increase maintenance energy requirements. One of the greatest hindrances to cattle performing in nonsummer months is mud.[38]

Windbreaks and Shelters

On average, cattle fed in the winter with wind protection have slightly better performance than cattle without wind protection.[6] In general, cold stress will stimulate intake; however, with less daylight in the winter combined with the cold conditions, cattle may not aggressively go to feeding areas, thus feed intake is not always increased. Under these conditions, windbreaks have been found to be useful, especially for heavyweight cattle. It is important to design windbreaks to keep snow out of the areas where cattle are held. Wind protection needs to be far enough away to prevent snow from dumping into the area holding the cattle.

New cattle coming into the feedlot and cattle 30 to 45 days from slaughter are most susceptible to cold stress.[36] They need shelter and/or bedding to maintain health and stay on feed. It is satisfactory to change to a higher-roughage diet when a snowstorm is imminent to minimize overeating or acidosis, but this change should not be made too aggressively. A more stable DMI can maintain a more stable rumen environment.

Recent interest has been shown in solid-floor confinement feedlot units, in which bedding is applied year-round in the pens on a weekly basis.[39] These units can cost 2 to 3 times more than traditional outside feedlot units and have shown promise for controlling the total amount of waste that has to be managed and for greater control of environmental factors. These units seem to have the greatest benefit in areas where surface drainage is poor, soil and winter drying conditions enhance mud build-up, and added wastewater generated from normal precipitation constitutes a disposal problem. It is becoming increasingly important that optimum cattle comfort be maintained not only for optimizing efficiency but also for enhancing consumer perceptions and acceptance. Keeping cattle dry, clean, and comfortable is critical for accomplishing this goal, whether in open lots or in more confined structures.

To enhance animal comfort in feedlot pens and other areas in the winter, the following guidelines can be used: (1) Facilities should be designed to properly drain water away from areas where animals normally accumulate. (2) Pushing snow out of pens (preferably after every storm) or at least to the low end of the facilities will minimize the effects of gradual melting and aid in drying out the resting areas. (3) Smooth out or knock down rough (frozen) surfaces that may impede access of feed and water. (4) Double the space allocation per animal. (The added space minimizes mud accumulation and allows for greater access to dry areas for animals to lie down.) (5) If animals are prone to getting wet, then use bedding and/or structures that provide wind protection while minimizing moisture effects.

Cattle, Cattle Handling, and Seasonal Differences

The effects of physical activity on BT are important if temperature is used as an indicator of health status. An elevated BT induced through physical activity or climatic factors could potentially provide false indicators of health status. Also, the BT of cattle fed high-energy diets in warm environments may already be elevated because of metabolic and climate-induced heat stress.[17,36]

In an experiment conducted in the winter in which cattle were moved approximately 500 m, tympanic temperatures (TT) were 0.8°C (38.3°C vs 39.1°C) and 0.7°C (38.6°C vs 39.3°C) greater ($P<.05$) in the morning and afternoon, respectively, than TT of the same cattle at corresponding times on days the cattle were not moved (**Fig. 3**). The process of moving cattle elevated TT immediately, most likely because of physical activity.[40] The TT during the nonmoved days remained low and in a fairly narrow temperature range. The time associated with the increase or peak in TT, as a result of moving, were 15 and 30 minutes in the morning and afternoon, respectively. Cattle TT returned to control (nonmoved day) TT levels 3.5 hours after peak TT were observed for both morning and afternoon moves. In summer, the increase in BT from handling can exceed 1°C for cattle with a mild disposition but can exceed 2°C for cattle that are easily excited.[41]

When cattle were exposed to hot conditions in the summer, TT display a greater range than when cattle were exposed to cold conditions in the winter. The maximum TT were greater ($P<.01$) and the minimum TT were lower ($P<.01$) in the summer than in the winter. Analysis of hourly data (see **Fig. 1**) indicated that the peak summer TT occurred around 1700 hours, whereas the peak winter TT are not as evident. Also, during hot environmental conditions, TT of dark or black-hided cattle are 0.5°C to 0.8°C greater than light or white-hided cattle from mid to late afternoon (**Fig. 4**). Cattle that are most susceptible to heat stress would, therefore, be black hided and cattle being full-fed a high-energy diet. Cattle nearly finished or carrying above-average body condition would also be subject to heat stress.

SUMMARY

Domestic livestock that are traditionally managed outdoors are particularly vulnerable not only to extreme environmental conditions but also to rapid changes in these conditions. Management and facility alternatives need to be considered to help these animals cope with adverse conditions. Manipulation of dietary ingredients, energy density, and intake may also be beneficial for livestock challenged by environmental

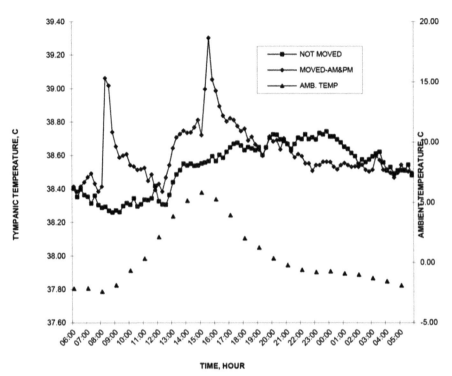

Fig. 3. TT of cattle moved through working facility. AMB, ambient temperature. (*Data from* Mader TL, Davis MS, Kreikemeier WM. Case study: tympanic temperature and behavior associated with moving feedlot cattle. Prof Anim Sci 2005;21:339–44.)

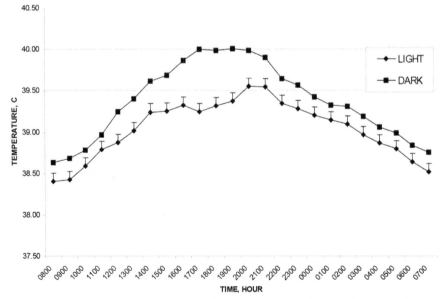

Fig. 4. TT of dark- versus light-hided cattle. (*From* Mader TL, Holt SM, Hahn GL, et al. Spiers. Feeding strategies for managing heat load in feedlot cattle. J Anim Sci 2002;80(9):2373–82; with permission.)

conditions. In addition, under hot conditions, high-volume water-holding devices and water availability is of upmost importance. Under cold conditions, maintaining facilities that prevent animals from getting wet/muddy is of upmost importance.

REFERENCES

1. Gaughan JB, Mader TL, Holt SM, et al. Assessing the heat tolerance of 17 beef cattle genotypes. Int J Biometeorol 2010;54:617–27.
2. Mader TL, Johnson LJ, Gaughan JB. A comprehensive index for assessing environmental stress in cattle. J Anim Sci 2010;88:2153–65.
3. Mader TL, Davis MS, Brown-Brandl T. Environmental factors influencing heat stress in feedlot cattle. J Anim Sci 2006;84:712–9.
4. Mader T, Griffin D, Hahn L. Managing feedlot heat stress. Univ. of Nebraska-Lincoln. NebGuide G00-1409-A. 2007. Available at: www.ianrpubs.unl.edu/epublic/pages/publicationD.jsp?publicationId=15. Accessed November 1, 2013.
5. Mader TL, Gaughan JB, Kreikemeier WM, et al. Behavioural effects of yearling grain-finished heifers exposed to differing environmental conditions and growth-promoting agents. Austr J Exp Agric 2008;48:1155–60.
6. Mader TL, Dahlquist JM, Gaughan JB. Wind protection effects and airflow patterns in outside feedlots. J Anim Sci 1997;75:26–36.
7. Gaughan JB, Mader TL, Holt SM, et al. A new heat load index for feedlot cattle. J Anim Sci 2008;86:226–34.
8. Gaughan JB, Bonner S, Loxton I, et al. Effect of shade on body temperature and performance of feedlot steers. J Anim Sci 2010;88:4056–67.
9. Brown-Brandl TM, Nienaber JA, Eigenberg RA, et al. Comparison of heat tolerance of feedlot heifers of different breeds. Livest Sci 2006;105:19–26.
10. Gaughan JB, Mader TL. Body temperature and respiratory dynamics in unshaded beef cattle. Int J Biometeorol 2014;58:1443–50.
11. Mader TL, Gaughan JB, Johnson LJ, et al. Tympanic temperature in confined beef cattle exposed to excessive heat load. Int J Biometeorol 2010;54:629–35.
12. Eigenberg RA, Brown-Brandl TM, Nienaber JA, et al. Dynamic response indicators of heat stress in shaded and non-shaded feedlot cattle, part 2: predictive relationships. Biosystems Eng 2005;91:111–8.
13. Mader TL, Holt SM, Hahn GL, et al. Feeding strategies for managing heat load in feedlot cattle. J Anim Sci 2002;80(9):2373–82.
14. Davis MS, Mader TL, Holt SM, et al. Strategies to reduce feedlot cattle heat stress: effects on tympanic temperature. J Anim Sci 2003;81:649–61.
15. Reinhardt CD, Brandt RT. Effect of morning vs evening feeding of limited-fed Holsteins during summer months. In: Kansas State Univ. Cattleman's Day Rep. Manhattan (KS): Kansas State Univ; 1994. p. 38–9.
16. Mader TL, Davis MS. Effect of management strategies on reducing heat stress of feedlot cattle: feed and water intake. J Anim Sci 2004;82:3077–87.
17. Mader TL, Gaughan JM, Young BA. Feedlot diet roughage level of Hereford cattle exposed to excessive heat load. Prof Anim Sci 1999;15:53–62.
18. Arias RA, Mader TL, Parkhurst AM. Effects of diet type and metabolizable energy intake level on tympanic temperature of steers fed during summer and winter seasons. J Anim Sci 2011;89:1574–80.
19. Gaughan JB, Mader TL. Effects of sodium chloride and fat supplementation on finishing steers exposed to hot and cold conditions. J Anim Sci 2009;87:612–21.
20. Savage D, Nolan J, Godwin I, et al. Importance of drinking water temperature for managing heat stress in sheep. Aust J Exp Ag 2008;48(7):1044–7.

21. Mader TL, Fell LR, McPhee MJ. Behavior response of non-Brahman cattle to shade in commercial feedlots. In: Proc. 5th Int. Livest. Envir. Symp. St. Joseph (MI): Amer. Soc. Agric. Eng.; 1997. p. 795–802.

22. Kelly CF, Bond TE, Ittner NR. Thermal design of livestock shades. Agr Eng 1950; 30:601–6.

23. Gaughan JB, Mader TL, Holt SM. Cooling and feeding strategies to reduce heat load of grain-fed beef cattle in intensive housing. Livest Sci 2008;113:226–33.

24. Mader TL, Dahlquist JM, Hahn GL, et al. Shade and wind barrier effects on summer-time feedlot cattle performance. J Anim Sci 1999;77:2065–72.

25. Sullivan ML, Cawdell-Smith AJ, Mader TL, et al. Effect of shade area on performance and welfare of short-fed feedlot cattle. J Anim Sci 2011;89:2911–25.

26. Hahn L, Mader T, Spiers D, et al. Heat wave impacts on feedlot cattle: considerations for improved environmental management. In: Proc. 6th Intl. Livest. Envir. Symp. St Joseph (MI): Amer. Soc. Agric. Eng; 2001. p. 129–30.

27. Mitlöhner JL, Morrow JW, Dailey SC, et al. Shade and water misting effects on behavior, physiology, performance, and carcass traits of heat-stressed feedlot cattle. J Anim Sci 2001;79:2327–35.

28. Mader TL. A tool for managing mud in feedlot pens. Intl. Symp. on Beef Cattle Welfare. Manhattan (KS): KSU; May 19–21, 2010.

29. Mader TL. Heat stress mitigation strategies – costs and benefits. Beef and dairy meeting. Mexicali, Mexico: University of Baja; October 2010. p. 6–10.

30. Mader TL. Impact of environmental stress on feedlot cattle. Proceedings of western section. Am Soc Anim Sci 2012;63:335–9.

31. Livestock Conservation Institute. Patterns of transit losses. Omaha (NE): Livestock Conservation Institute; 1970.

32. NOAA. Livestock hot weather stress. Operations manual letter C-31-76. Kansas City (MO): NOAA; 1976.

33. Hubbard KG, Stooksbury DE, Hahn GL, et al. A climatological perspective on feedlot cattle performance and mortality related to the temperature-humidity index. J Prod Agric 1999;12:650–3.

34. Chichester M, Mader TL. Heat stress – What you should know to make livestock shows a success. Univ. of Nebraska-Lincoln. NebGuide G2121. 2012. Available at: http://www.ianrpubs.unl.edu/epublic/live/g2121/build/. Accessed November 1, 2013.

35. NRC. Nutrient requirements of beef cattle. 7th edition. Washington, DC: Natl. Acad. Press; 2000.

36. Mader TL. Environmental stress in confined beef cattle. J Anim Sci 2003;81(E Suppl 2):E110–9.

37. Mader TL, Colgan SL. Pen density and straw bedding during feedlot finishing. Nebraska Beef Report MP90. Lincoln (NE): Univ. of Nebraska-Lincoln; 2007. p. 43–6.

38. Mader TL. Mud effects on feedlot cattle. Nebraska beef report MP94. Lincoln (NE): Univ. of Nebraska-Lincoln; 2011. p. 82–3.

39. Pastoor JW, Loy DD, Trenkle A, et al. Comparing fed cattle performance in open lot and bedded confinement feedlot facilities. Prof Anim Scientist 2012;28:410–6.

40. D'Allaire S, DeRoth L. Physiological responses to treadmill exercise and ambient temperature in normal and malignant hyperthermia susceptible pigs. Can J Vet Res 1986;50:78.

41. Brown-Brandl TM. Heat stress in feedlot cattle. CAB reviews: perspectives in agriculture, veterinary science, nutrition and natural resources, vol. 3. Boston (MA): Cabi; 2008. p. 16.

Animal Health Equipment Management

David N. Rethorst, DVM

KEYWORDS

• Animals • Health • Equipment • Management

KEY POINTS

- Establishing and following protocols during processing is required to ensure producing a safe product that is free of defects and residues.
- In this age of increasing production transparency, overall cleanliness of equipment and facilities is important not only from a food safety standpoint but many view these as an overall indicator of attention to detail in the entire production system.
- Ensuring that needles are changed, implant guns are managed properly, vaccine is handled in an acceptable manner, and proper chute operation occurs is essential.

Sanitation and proper use of animal health equipment used in processing and treatment of beef cattle should be a primary concern of both veterinarians and producers to ensure product quality and safety. Bacterial and viral nosocomial infections can occur in cattle as a result of improper sanitation of facilities and equipment.[1] Zoonotic illnesses can occur in animal caregivers as a result of improper sanitation. Environmental contaminants such as *Escherichia coli* and *Salmonella* spp are spread between cattle by improperly sanitized equipment.[1] Improper injection location, changing of needles, and inadequate cleaning of syringes can lead to injection site blemishes, scar tissue, or bacterial infections, which affect the quality and safety of the end product.[2,3]

BIOSECURITY: ISOLATION, TRAFFIC CONTROL, AND SANITATION

The goal of a biosecurity plan is to prevent or control cross-contamination of feces, urine, saliva, and so forth between animals to prevent or control the spread of pathogens between animals.[4] This plan should consider direct as well as indirect animal contact. Indirect contact considerations include animal to feed transmission and animal to equipment transmission. The 3 components of biosecurity are isolation, traffic control, and sanitation.

The author has nothing to disclose.
Department of Diagnostic Medicine and Pathobiology, Beef Cattle Institute, Kansas State University, College of Veterinary Medicine, Trotter Hall, Room 1, Manhattan, KS 66502, USA
E-mail address: drethorst@vet.ksu.edu

Vet Clin Food Anim 31 (2015) 259–267
http://dx.doi.org/10.1016/j.cvfa.2015.03.009

Isolation is the most important step in disease control, because it prevents direct contact between diseased or potentially infected cattle and healthy cattle. Preventing commingling of new cattle and existing groups of cattle is crucial to an effective biosecurity plan. Facilities used to segregate cattle should be cleaned between groups and disinfected if deemed appropriate.

Traffic control includes all traffic on an operation, animals, people, and vehicles or equipment. Animals to consider include all domesticated animals as well as rodents, birds, and other wildlife. Fecal contamination of feedstuffs such as silage or ground hay can be controlled by limiting traffic to the silage pit and hay pile to the loader designated to load feed. Another major concern of traffic control is limiting rendering truck access to an area of the yard that is away from all cattle and feeding activities.

Sanitation refers not only to the disinfection of people and equipment entering an operation but the cleanliness of people and equipment on the operation. Prevention of fecal–oral contamination is the primary goal of sanitation. Balling guns and drench guns are of primary concern for disinfecting between animals. Before disinfection, the equipment should be cleaned with soap and hot water at the end of each day and stored in a dry area.

Another major biosecurity consideration is loaders that are used to load feedstuffs. If these loaders are used for handling manure, dead cattle, or other nonfeedstuff products, they should be cleaned and disinfected before loading feedstuffs. Processing and treatment areas should be cleaned at the end of each day. This strategy reduces the likelihood of fecal–oral contamination not only of the cattle but of the caregivers as well.

The first step in sanitation is the removal of organic matter, primarily feces. Any blood or saliva present should also be removed. Disinfection should follow this cleaning. Physical contact between the disinfectant and proper contact time are crucial to ensure proper disinfection. The selected disinfectant should kill a broad spectrum of bacteria, viruses, protozoa, fungi, and spores.[5] Other selection considerations include safety to both humans and animal, effect on equipment (corrosiveness), effect on environment, and cost (**Tables 1** and **2**).

VETERINARY EQUIPMENT SANITATION

Equipment used for processing and treating cattle should be cleaned and disinfected daily, after use. If this equipment becomes grossly contaminated with feces or other material while being used, it should be cleaned immediately.

Equipment such as balling guns and drench guns should be thoroughly cleaned at the end of each day and stored in a clean, dry environment. Disinfecting this equipment between animals is recommended. The disinfectant solution should be changed when it becomes cloudy or visibly contaminated to maintain effectiveness. Increased morbidity and mortality in feeder cattle have been associated with improper sanitation of this equipment in a feedyard hospital system having a high prevalence of *Salmonella* infection.[1] Cohort cattle that did not go through the hospital system were found to have zero prevalence for *Salmonella* spp.

Disinfecting of blood-contaminated equipment between animals is essential. This strategy reduces the risk of transmission for pathogens such as bovine virus diarrhea virus, bovine leukosis virus, and various other blood-borne pathogens. Disinfection also reduces bacterial contamination and risk of disease transmitted animal to animal. This equipment includes dehorners, castration equipment, and various instruments used for minor surgical procedures. Thorough cleaning is necessary, followed by storage in a clean, dry area. Banding castration equipment should be kept free of feces

Table 1
Disinfectant selection table

Compound	Chlorine 0.01%–5%	Iodine Iodophor 0.5%–5%	Chlorhexidine 0.05%–0.5%	Alcohol 70%–95%	Oxidizing 0.2%–3%	Phenol 0.2%–3%	Quaternary Ammonium 0.1%–2%	Aldehyde 1%–2%
Examples	Clorox	Tincture/provodine	Nolvasan		Vikron S	Lysol	Roccal-D	Wavicide
Bactericidal	Good	Good	Very good	Good	Good	Good	Good	Very good
Viricidal	Very good	Good	Fair	Good	Excellent	Fair	Fair	Very good
Envelope viruses	Yes	Yes	Yes	Yes	Yes	Yes	Yes	Yes
Nonenvelope viruses	Yes	Yes	No	No	Yes	No	No	Yes
Bacterial spores	Fair	Fair	Poor	Fair	Fair	Poor	Poor	Good
Fungicidal	Good	Good	Fair	Fair	Fair	Good	Fair	Good
Effective in organic matter	Poor	Fair	Fair	Poor	Fair	Good	Fair	Good
Inactivated by soap	No	Yes/no	Yes	No	No	No	Yes	No
Effective in hard water	Yes	No	Yes	Yes	Yes	Yes	No	Yes
Contact time (min)	5–30	10–30	5–10	1–30	10–30	10–30	10–30	10–600
Residual activity	Poor	Poor	Good	Poor	Poor	Poor	Fair	Fair

Adapted from Bek TJ, Griffin D, Kennedy J. Selection and use of disinfectants. NebGuide G1410: Cooperative Extension, Institute of Agriculture and Natural Resources, University of Nebraska-Lincoln; 2000 and Data from Refs.[5–9]

Table 2
Cattle viruses with and without envelopes

Virus	Envelope	Virus	Envelope	Virus	Envelope
Bluetongue	No	Malignant catarrhal fever	Yes	PI3	Yes
Rotavirus	No	Enteric coronavirus	Yes	Rabies	Yes
Papillomatosis	No	Respiratory coronavirus	Yes	Herpes mammillitis	Yes
Foot-and-mouth disease	No	Bovine virus diarrhea	Yes	Cowpox	Yes
Leukemia	Yes	Bovine respiratory syncytial virus	Yes	Pseudocowpox	Yes
Papular stomatitis	Yes	Infectious bovine rhinotracheitis/ infectious pustular vulvovaginitis	Yes	Lumpy skin disease	Yes
Vesicular stomatitis	Yes				

From Bek TJ, Griffin D, Kennedy J. Selection and use of disinfectants. NebGuide G1410: Cooperative Extension, Institute of Agriculture and Natural Resources, University of Nebraska-Lincoln; 2000.

and other gross contaminates between animals. Thorough cleaning at the end of the day is appropriate.

Cleaning and disinfection of obstetric equipment is an often neglected area. All obstetric equipment, calf pullers, chains, straps, head snares, and so forth should be thoroughly cleaned and disinfected after each use. If straps are being used rather than chains, extra attention should be given to making sure that the strap is clean and dry before storing. Chains should be allowed to dry completely before storing to prevent rusting.

One of the most consistent, positive returns on investment procedures in the cattle industry is the use of growth-promoting implants. For this practice to be effective, care must be taken to ensure that it is performed properly. Implant guns should be thoroughly washed with detergent and hot water after each use and allowed to dry. It is essential that the needles on these guns are sharp. If needles become dull or burred, they should be discarded rather than attempting to sharpen them. The ear should be free of feces and other gross contamination. If not, the ear should be cleaned with a disinfectant solution before placing the implant. A sponge or paint roller in a disinfectant solution should be available to clean the implant needle after each animal is implanted. If the needle skips off the ear, the needle should be disinfected before another attempt to implant is made.

CARE AND CLEANING OF VETERINARY VACCINE SYRINGES

Inadequate care and cleaning of syringes used for routine vaccination of livestock can be associated with localized swelling and infection after vaccination.[2] Swellings involving the injection site are common, particularly when vaccines such as clostridial vaccines are given subcutaneously. The subcutaneous use of oil-adjuvanted vaccines also results in swelling of the injection site. If these swellings do not subside in a short period, if they become larger than a small hen's egg, or if they become fluid filled, they may be infected and should be examined.[2]

Proper cleaning of syringes begins with using hot water, soap, and a brush to clean the external surface and working mechanism of the syringe. Care should be taken to keep soap away from the luer tip of the syringe. After cleaning the external components, rinse the internal components with distilled or deionized water that is warmer than 82.2°C (180°F) by drawing the water into the syringe and squirting it out several times.[2] All syringes, whether pistol grip repeaters or continuous feed syringes with vinyl tubing and vent spikes, can be cleaned in this manner. Soap and disinfectant should not be used on the internal components of syringes. Remove as much water as possible from the syringe and allow it to cool before use, because heat inactivates modified live viral vaccines. Some syringes may need to be disassembled to adequately clean them. Disassembly should be performed on a clean work surface followed by cleaning the components with hot tap water, avoiding the use of soap or disinfectant. If syringes are physically contaminated enough to require disassembly for cleaning, they should be boiled for 5 minutes in deionized or distilled water. Plastic, continuous feed syringes can be sanitized after cleaning, if necessary. The syringe and tubing should be filled with distilled water and wrapped in multiple layers of paper towels. After soaking the paper towels in water, the syringe is placed in an unclosed zip-lock bag. This bag is placed in a microwave oven for 5 minutes using the high setting. Care should be taken that the paper towels do not dry out during this process. Syringes should be individually microwaved when using this method. After the syringes are removed from the microwave, any water remaining in them should be squirted out and the syringe allowed to cool before using.

Syringes should be reassembled while hot, using lubricant such as vegetable oil spray on the rubber plunger.[2] Others recommend using the first draw of vaccine as the lubricant, thus avoiding silicone, mineral oil, or Vaseline.[10] There does not seem to be a consensus as to what is acceptable (nonviricidal) in regard to syringe lubricant, because still others recommend the use of silicone or Vaseline.[11] This is an area that warrants further investigation.

Once assembled, the syringe should be rinsed several times with water warmer than 180°F. After cooling, the syringes should be stored in a clean, dry environment, such as a new zip-lock bag that is placed in a freezer. Syringes should be allowed to warm to room temperature before filling with vaccine. Warming the syringes by artificial means may result in hot spots in the syringes, which have the potential to damage the vaccine.

Syringes should be labeled to ensure that the same product goes in each syringe every time cattle are worked. This strategy eliminates the possibility of trace amounts of a vaccine or pharmaceutical remaining in a syringe and having a detrimental effect on the next product in the syringe. It also ensures that syringes are not filled with the wrong product during processing.

TRANSFER NEEDLE MANAGEMENT

Transfer needles should be cleaned in a manner similar to syringes, after using a stylet to remove rubber plugs from the needle, using hot water without soap or disinfectant. Once cleaned, there are several methods that can be used to ensure that the needles are sterile. These methods include[2]

1. Boiling in distilled water for 5 minutes. After cooling, the needles should be stored in a clean, dust-free container.
2. Microwaving the needles in a cup filled with distilled water. Use the high setting to bring the water to a boil. Once the water boils, continue for 1 minute. Be sure the needles are completely covered with water during the entire process. Once again, the needles should be stored in a clean, dust-free container after cooling.

3. Wrap the needles in several layers of paper towels. Soak the paper towels in water and place in a zip-lock bag. Place the unclosed zip-lock bag in a microwave for 2 minutes using the high setting. The paper towels should remain wet during the process. Store appropriately when cool.
4. Autoclaving works well if such equipment is available. The clean needles are placed in a 12-mL disposable syringe case or multiple needles in a 20-mL syringe case. The cap is held in place with autoclave tape. After autoclaving, the syringe cases work well for clean, dust-free storage.

NEEDLE SELECTION AND MANAGEMENT

The size of needles used for processing and treatment of cattle should be adjusted according to cattle size, viscosity of product injected, route of administration, and type of restraint to be used (**Table 3**). Use the smallest needle possible to easily administer the product, yet large enough to prevent the needle from bending or breaking off in the animal. The use of disposable needles is recommended, because they are sterile and are sharp. Using steel needles that are reusable is discouraged, because they are difficult to sterilize and keep sharp. Improper needle management results in injection site lesions that requires trimming during harvest or fabrication.[12]

Needles should be changed before they become dull, preferably every 10 to 15 head. In addition, they should be changed immediately if the needle bends, becomes contaminated with feces, dirt, or chemicals, or if the needle point is damaged. In herds that are known to be infected with pathogens that are blood borne, consideration should be given to changing needles after each animal. Never use a needle that is bent, because this increases the likelihood that the needle will break off in the animal being injected. It is considered an emergency situation when a needle breaks off in an animal. If this occurs, great effort should be made to find the needle immediately. If the needle cannot be found, the animal should be identified to be checked later. An animal that is known to have a broken needle in it should not be marketed for human consumption.

The best method for disposal of used needles is the collection of needles in a biohazard sharps container, which should be disposed of by a biomedical disposal company. An alternative disposal method is collecting the needles in a plastic jug or bucket and filling the bucket with cement powder and water before sealing it and disposing of it in a landfill. Used needles should never be disposed of individually in

Table 3
Needle selection guide

	Route of Administration								
	SQ (0.5–0.75 inch Needle)			IV (1.5 inch Needle)			IM (1–1.5 inch Needle)		
	Cattle Weight			Cattle Weight			Cattle Weight		
Injectable viscosity	<300	300–700	>700	<300	300–700	>700	<300	300–700	>700
Thin (gauge) Example: Saline	18	18–16	16	18–16	16		16–14	20–18	18–16	18–16
Thick (gauge) Example: Oxytetracycline	18–16	18–16	16	16	16–14	16–14	18	16	16

Select the needle to fit the cattle size (the smallest practical size without bending).
Adapted from Beef quality assurance. Best management practices–prevention and processing. National Beef Quality Assurance manual. National Cattlemen's Beef Association, Centennial, CO.

the daily trash. State law should be checked if one is unsure of the legalities of needle disposal in one's local area.

VACCINE STORAGE AND HANDLING

For vaccines to induce adequate immunity, they must be shipped, stored, and handled in a proper manner, including the handling that occurs during administration. Although this factor is especially important for modified live vaccines, it applies to all vaccines whether modified live virus, killed virus, or a bacterin toxoid.

Refrigerators used to store animal health products come in all shapes and sizes, ranging from minirefrigerators to household-type refrigerators to glass-front display coolers. Many of the household-type refrigerators are used refrigerators purchased for the sole purpose of storage of animal health products. These refrigerators are found in a variety of places from the barn, to the shop, to the mudroom, or even the kitchen. Retailers such as feed stores and veterinary clinics are another common location for refrigerators used to store animal health products.

Two studies funded by state Beef Quality Assurance programs have evaluated how well these refrigerators cool. The first study evaluated 191 refrigerators.[13] Of these refrigerators, only 51 (26.7%) operated within the desired temperature range greater than 95% of the time over the 48-hour test period. Thirty-eight (19.9%) operated at the correct temperature 66% to 95% of the time, whereas 34 (17.8%) operated properly 36% to 65% of the time and 23 (12.0%) were in the correct range 5% to 35% of the time. The remaining 45 refrigerators (23.6%) operated at the desired temperature less than 5% of the time. Nearly 43% of these 191 refrigerators were greater than 10 years old. The second study evaluated 176 refrigerators.[3] Producer refrigerators accounted for 129 of the 176, whereas 47 were feedstore or veterinary clinic refrigerators. Forty (31%) of the 129 refrigerators operated at the correct temperature greater than 95% of the time, with another 19 (14.5%), operating properly 66% to 95% of the time. Forty-three (33.3%) were at the correct temperature less than 5% of the time. The retail coolers were similar, in that 16 (34%) were at the correct temperature greater than 95% of the time. Seven (14.9%) operated properly 66% to 95% of the time and 10 (21.3%), were at the correct temperature 36% to 65% of the time. Eight (17%) were found to be at the proper temperature less than 5% of the time.

The desired temperature range as defined for these studies was 2°C to 7°C (35°F–45°F), which is the temperature range commonly recommended by the pharmaceutical industry. Temperatures lower than 2°C (35°F) can be more detrimental than temperatures higher than 7°C (45°F) because of antigen–adjuvant separation.[9] Temperatures higher than 7°C (45°F) are particularly detrimental to modified live vaccines.

Location of the refrigerators in this study seemed to account for a portion of the fluctuation of the temperature. Those refrigerators that were in a controlled environment maintained proper temperature in a more acceptable manner than did those that were located in an uninsulated building.

An interesting observation in these studies was the number of outdated products and open bottles of product, including modified live viral vaccine, that were found in the refrigerators evaluated. Of the 1800 products found in producer refrigerators in the first survey,[13] 11.8% were outdated and 29.3% were open. The second survey[14] found nearly 2260 products in the refrigerators, of which 20.5% were expired and 27.2% were open.

A summary of these 2 refrigerator studies includes the following:

1. Keep a thermometer in the refrigerator so that temperature can be monitored.
2. Do not use minirefrigerators for long-term storage.

3. Keep the refrigerator in a controlled environment.
4. Regular cleaning of the coil and compressor are essential, particularly if the refrigerator is located in a barn or processing shed.
5. Refrigerators that do not maintain temperature between 2°C and 7°C (35°F – 45°F) should be replaced.

When vaccine is taken from the refrigerator to chute-side, it should be stored in a cooler box with freezer packs. This strategy not only keeps the vaccine cool but provides for storage of the vaccine out of direct sunlight once it has been mixed. No more modified live viral vaccine should be mixed than is anticipated will be used in 1 hour. Open vaccine, whether modified live or killed, should be stored in the cooler box unless syringes are being filled. Modified live vaccine that has been mixed should be discarded when the cattle have been processed, because of the short life of the vaccine ($\leq$1 hour).

Care should be taken to ensure that a used needle never enters a bottle of vaccine. A used needle can contaminate the remainder of the vaccine, resulting in injection site blemishes. The importance of cleanliness during processing is shown by the fact that dried nasal secretions from a calf persistently infected with bovine virus diarrhea (BVD) virus on the rubber stopper of a vaccine bottle transmitted BVD virus to a seronegative calf.[1]

The storage environment of nonrefrigerated pharmaceutical products such as antibiotics, anthelmintics, and topical insecticides should be considered. These products should be protected from freezing and heat, because either can cause damage to the product. If the rubber stoppers on stored bottles of product are damaged enough to not seal the bottle, the product may deteriorate because of exposure to air. These bottles should be capped in some manner, such as a roll-on rubber stopper, to prevent exposure of the product to air.

HYDRAULIC CHUTE MANAGEMENT

The operating pressure and thus the operating speed of a hydraulic chute are set by the manufacturer and should not be changed. Although this pressure setting varies between manufacturers, the basic guideline is 272 kg (600 lb) of squeeze pressure measured at the bottom of the squeeze panel drop gates using a pressure bar between the 2 squeeze panels (D.D. Griffin, personal communication, 2015). For this pressure to be accurate, the distance between the bottom of the squeeze panels should be slightly narrower than the distance between the squeeze panels at the bottom of the drop gates (simulate shoulder width vs stance width).

The chute operator should always use 2 hands on the controls. This technique allows for smoother handling of the cattle and reduces the bruising that can be associated with processing. Before cattle enter the chute, the distance between the bottoms of the squeeze panels should be observed. This distance should be approximately the stance width for the class of cattle being processed. If this distance is too narrow, excessive pressure will be applied to the animal when the squeeze is applied. As the operator prepares to let cattle enter the chute, the tailgate is opened with the squeeze slightly closed and the headgate open no wider than the animal's shoulders.

As the animal proceeds into the chute, it is slowed with the squeeze panels to prevent it from slamming into the headgate. The headgate is closed, the tailgate closed and then, if necessary the squeeze panels. When releasing the animal, the headgate should be opened first, then the squeeze released. When this sequence is followed, the cattle tend to move forward, without the use of an electrical prod. If the squeeze is released before opening the headgate, the cattle tend to back up, necessitating prod use in many instances. The use of low-stress handling practices before the animal enters the chute can reduce the risk of injury and problems associated with hydraulic chute use.

SUMMARY

Proper health equipment management requires significant attention to detail. Establishing and following protocols during processing (eg, cleaning and disinfecting equipment at the end of the work day) is required to ensure a safe product that is free of defects and residues. In this age of increasing production transparency, overall cleanliness of equipment and facilities is important not only from a food safety standpoint but many view these as an overall indicator of attention to detail in the entire production system. Therefore, ensuring that needles are changed, implant guns are managed properly, vaccine is handled in an acceptable manner, and proper chute operation occurs is essential.

REFERENCES

1. Thomson DU. Feedlot hospital management. In: Anderson DE, Rings DM, editors. Current veterinary therapy: food animal practice. St. Louis (MO): Saunders; 2009. p. 678–81.
2. Griffin DD, Ensley S, Smith DR, et al. Care of veterinary vaccine syringes. NebGuide G02-1443-A. Lincoln (NE): Cooperative Extension, Institute of Agriculture and Natural Resources, University of Nebraska-Lincoln; 2002.
3. Best management practices–prevention and processing. National Beef Quality Assurance manual. Centennial (CO): National Cattlemen's Beef Association; 2008. p. 13–69.
4. Buhman M, Dewell G, Griffin D, et al. Biosecurity basics for cattle operations and good management practices (GMP) for controlling infectious diseases. NebGuide G1411. Lincoln (NE): Cooperative Extension, Institute of Agriculture and Natural Resources, University of Nebraska-Lincoln; 2000. p. 2007.
5. Dvorak G, Roth J, Amass S, et al. Disinfection 101. Ames (IA): Center for Food Security and Public Health, Iowa State University; 2008.
6. Wickstrom ML. Overview of antiseptics and disinfectants. Whitehouse Station (NJ): Merck Veterinary Manual; 2012.
7. Boothe HW. Antiseptics and disinfectants. Vet Clin North Am Small Anim Pract 1998;28:233–48.
8. Cleaning and disinfection of environmental surfaces. Health Care Health and Safety Association of Ontario; 2004.
9. Geering WA, Penrith ML, Nyakahuma D, et al. Manual on procedures for disease eradication by stamping out. Rome (IT): Food and Agriculture Organization of the United Nations; 2001.
10. Thrift TA, Hersom MJ, Irsik M, et al. Florida cow-calf and stocker beef safety and quality assurance handbook: quality control points. AN 173. Gainesville (FL): University of Florida; 2006. p. 2013.
11. Pence M. Vaccine handling and syringe care. Athens (GA): University of Georgia College of Veterinary Medicine; 2005.
12. Dexter DR, Cowman GL, Morgan JB, et al. Incidence of injection-site blemishes in beef top sirloin butts. J Anim Sci 1994;72:824–7.
13. Troxel TR, Barham BL. Case study: the temperature variability of refrigerators storing animal health products. Professional Animal Scientist 2009;25:202–6.
14. Fife TE, Troxel TR, Barham BL, et al. Case study: handling and management of animal health products by Idaho producers and retailers. Professional Animal Scientist 2013;29:313–20.

Beef Quality Assurance in Feedlots

Robert A. Smith, DVM, MS[a], Daniel U. Thomson, DVM, PhD[b],*,
Tiffany L. Lee, DVM, MSc, MS[b]

KEYWORDS

• Feedlot • BQA • Cattle handling • Drug use • Injection sites

KEY POINTS

• The Beef Quality Assurance (BQA) program was written by beef producers and veterinarians for beef producers and veterinarians.
• The program has continued to evolve from its starting point of antibiotic residue avoidance to include animal handling, cattle comfort, food safety, and much more.
• Providing guidance to producers and veterinarians on best management practices allows the beef industry to be transparent and open to the beef consumer about the practices used on cattle.
• Veterinarians are key components to helping producers implement BQA in their beef operations.

INTRODUCTION

Veterinarians and cattlemen have long recognized the need to properly care for cattle. Historically, beef production practices fell under the "animal husbandry" umbrella and focused primarily on feeding, breeding, and disease management. As time progressed, consumers became more interested in specific beef production practices, ranging from antimicrobial use, growth enhancement, food-borne illness, and cattle care and well-being. This, as well as advancing beef production technologies and knowledge, guided significant changes in beef production practices over the past 30 years.

In the early 1980s, the beef cattle industry began exploring ways to assure consumers that beef is a safe product. One of the first steps was to establish a relationship between the US Department of Agriculture Food Safety Inspection Service and the beef industry to develop the Pre-Harvest Beef Safety Production Program. This was key to the later development of the Beef Quality Assurance (BQA) program.[1]

The authors have nothing to disclose.
[a] CattleTec Veterinary Services, PLLC, Veterinary Research and Consulting Services, LLC, 3404 Live Oak Lane, Stillwater, OK 74075, USA; [b] Beef Cattle Institute, Kansas State University, 101 Trotter Hall, Manhattan, KS 66506, USA
* Corresponding author.
E-mail address: dthomson@vet.k-state.edu

Vet Clin Food Anim 31 (2015) 269–281
http://dx.doi.org/10.1016/j.cvfa.2015.03.008   vetfood.theclinics.com
0749-0720/15/$ – see front matter © 2015 Elsevier Inc. All rights reserved.

Over the next few decades, the beef industry adopted self-regulating programs without additional governmental regulation to provide greater assurances to consumers that best production practices were animal-friendly and that beef products were of the highest quality. Various BQA programs were expanded to include truckers, auction markets, cow-calf producers, stocker operators, feedlots, packers, and dairies. Education of stakeholders in the production chain was the cornerstone, with educational materials developed in cooperation with the National Cattlemen's Beef Association, state cattlemen's associations, beef councils, university extension, nutritionists, animal behaviorists, and veterinarians.

More recently, the beef industry has developed the framework for individuals and businesses involved in beef production to become BQA certified.[2] At the same time, assessment guides were developed for cow-calf, stocker, and feedlot owners and/or managers to assess compliance with BQA principles.[3] Third-party audits are performed to ensure that beef production practices are followed.

Throughout its history, the goal of BQA has been simple: improve the quality of beef to provide consumers with what they want. When accomplished, this improves consumer demand, optimizes the well-being of cattle, and increases the likelihood of profit for beef producers.

INJECTION-SITE LESIONS

Injectable animal health products for beef cattle are more commonly used than those administered orally or topically. Until the early 1990s, the intramuscular (IM) route of administration was more common than the subcutaneous (SC) route. Research has shown that any animal health product administered IM can cause an injection-site lesion in muscle tissue. The lesions are also called injection-site scars, blemishes, or defects. A Colorado State University study demonstrated that administration of clostridial vaccine or an antibiotic at branding (50 days of age) or weaning (200 days of age) resulted in injection-site lesions that persisted until harvest at about 14 months of age.[4]

Another study evaluated the incidence, severity, amount of tissue affected, and effect on histology when the top sirloin butt (biceps femoris and gluteus medius muscles) and outside round (biceps femoris muscle) were injected IM with various animal health products. Weaning-age beef calves were randomly injected with10 mL sterile saline, 2 mL modified-live virus vaccine (Bovi-Shield 4), 5 mL inactivated virus vaccine with oil adjuvant (Vira Shield 5), 5 mL 7-way clostridial bacterin-toxoid (Clostridial 7-way), 5 mL vitamin ADE (Vital E-A+D), 8.8 mL (average) aqueous antibiotic (Naxcel), 10 mL tylosin (Tylosin Injection), or10 mL long-acting oxytetracycline (Liquamycin LA-200). The contralateral noninjected subprimals served as controls. Products were administered IM using a 16 gauge, one and one-half inch (38.1 mm) needle. Calves were fed in a commercial feedlot and harvested in a commercial packing plant after 178 days on feed.[5,6]

Visible injection-site lesions were observed in 7.1% to 100% in both the top sirloin butts (average incidence 55.8%) and outside rounds (average incidence 54.5%), depending on the product injected. Subprimals with visible lesions had higher ($P<.001$) mean shear force values (Warner-Bratzler shear device) and more variation in tenderness than noninjected controls. Subprimals that were injected but had no visible lesions had higher ($P<.001$) shear force values and more ($P<.01$) variation in tenderness than control primal cuts. The investigators concluded that IM administration of all compounds resulted in unacceptable muscle tissue quality, specifically a decrease in tenderness.[5,6]

Research and the high incidence of visible injection-site lesions in top sirloin butts observed during audits at steak-cutting operations provided strong evidence of the causes of injection-site damage and served as the impetus to change the way animal health products were administered to cattle, which in turn improved beef quality by reducing defects.

GUIDELINES FOR USE OF INJECTABLE PRODUCTS

Veterinarians typically spend more time in feedlots than other consultants or advisors. As such, veterinarians are well positioned to train and observe animal-care personnel when cattle are processed or treated for illness. Written protocols should provide product administration details and, when combined with training and periodic assessments, result in a high likelihood of BQA compliance. Almost all injectable products have the labeled option for SC administration. When the choice of SC or IM is offered, the SC route should be used to avoid muscle tissue damage. If a product is labeled only for IM use, administer it in the neck and never exceed 10 mL IM per injection site. There are no restrictions on the volume of SC injections other than indicated by the product label.[7] For example, the enrofloxacin (Baytril) label allows up to 20 mL per SC injection site whereas florfenicol (Nuflor) limits the volume to 10 mL at each SC injection site. All injectable medications and vaccines should be given in front of the shoulders, never in the rump or back leg. Multiple injection sites should be separated by at least a hand-width.[7]

Good restraint is essential for proper injection of pharmaceuticals and vaccines. Excessive animal movement can result in unpredicted movement of the needle, which can cause tissue damage or unnecessary pain in the animal. This strongly suggests that cattle should not be injected when trapped behind a gate or while crowded in the narrow lead-up alley (snake) behind the chute. Instead, cattle should be restrained in a chute with a headgate and side squeeze that limits mobility. The operator should catch the animal in the chute so that there is ample neck area for injections. Typically this is accomplished by catching the animal just behind the ears with the headgate.[8]

Needle selection is an important component of BQA. First, needles should be high quality to minimize the risk of needles breaking off in the animal and to remain sharp to make skin penetration easier. Needles should be changed after every 10 to 15 head, sooner if the needle becomes dull, burred, or soiled. It may be necessary to change needles more often if there is risk of blood-borne diseases.[8,9]

In most cases, a 16-gauge needle is suitable for giving injections to beef cattle; the needle is small enough to minimize risk of leak-back of product and to cause minimal discomfort to the animal but large enough to resist breaking off. A one-half to five-eighths inch (12.7–15.88 mm) length needle is usually sufficient to administer animal health products by the SC route, although the BQA Guidelines offer the choices of one-half to three-fourths inch (12.7–19.05 mm) for SC products, and one to one and one-half inch (25.4–38.1 mm) needles to administer products by the IM route.[8,9]

Veterinarians should provide a detailed written protocol for managing an animal with a broken needle. When this occurs, immediate action should be taken to remove the needle with forceps or by pressing the needle back through the skin. If unsuccessful, the injection site should be marked and a tag denoting "broken needle" should be placed in the ear. A veterinarian might be able to surgically retrieve the broken needle but, if the needle is not recovered, the animal must never be allowed to enter marketing channels.[7]

The angle of needle insertion is critical for proper SC administration of health products. Although a short needle is recommended, IM deposition of the drug or vaccine can occur if the needle is inserted at a 90° angle. Therefore, a needle angle approximating 30° is more likely to achieve the BQA goal of SC administration. "Tenting" of the skin, pulling the skin away from underlying tissues, can result in more accurate administration of vaccines or pharmaceuticals in the SC space. A 1-handed technique for administering products SC is effective when the correct angle of needle insertion is used.[8]

Ongoing monitoring and training will ensure that injections are given according to BQA guidelines. Veterinarians should examine injection sites during necropsy. Examination provides backup evidence that BQA guidelines are or are not being followed. In addition, injection site maps should be maintained to document where products were administered if injection site lesions are discovered. Records should include the name of the animal health products, route of administration, location, volume, serial number, and a daily statement verifying that no needles were broken off in the animals.

JUDICIOUS USE OF DRUGS IN CATTLE

Veterinarians have taken the oath to "use my scientific knowledge and skills for the benefit of society through the protection of animal health and welfare, the prevention and relief of animal suffering, the conservation of animal resources, the promotion of public health, and the advancement of medical knowledge."[10] Pharmaceuticals, vaccines, and chemicals are used for prevention and treatment of disease in feedlot cattle, to reduce animal suffering, and to enhance performance. The use of these tools, along with animal husbandry, has a positive impact on both production and well-being.

Veterinarians are charged with the responsibility for judicious use of animal health products in feedlot cattle because of professional responsibility to ensure prudent use of animal health products as well as state and federal laws and regulations. A veterinarian-client-patient relationship (VCPR) is essential to meet this obligation. According to the American Association of Bovine Practitioners (AABP) VCPR Guidelines, it is crucial that there is mutual agreement between the veterinarian and client that a VCPR exists, that there is a designated veterinarian of record, there are clear relationships with other veterinarians and consultants, written treatment protocols are provided, written or electronic treatment records are maintained, and drugs are prescribed or dispensed in a legal and ethical manner.[11]

Veterinarians must be familiar with the feedlot's operations so they can develop protocols for prevention and treatment of disease. This includes making timely visits to the feedlot, diagnostics, records analysis, and through interaction and training of caretakers. Protocols should be developed for use by management and feedlot employees. These should include definitions of conditions or diseases; clinical signs; guidelines for making treatment decisions; treatment regimens; and proper storage, handling, and administration of animal health products.[12] Detailed protocols and consistent oversight and training of feedlot employees help prevent protocol deviation or misuse of drugs. It is especially important to train feedlot employees on observing proper preharvest withdrawal times and maintaining electronic or written treatment records. These records should be kept for 3 years to be compliant with BQA guidelines and meet or exceed state and federal laws.

Prescribing or dispensing of drugs to feedlot clients must be done in accordance with state and federal laws. The first Federal Food and Drug Act in the United States was passed in 1906, and numerous laws have been passed since then to regulate drugs, vaccines, and chemicals.[13] Currently, the most relevant laws and regulations governing prescribing or dispensing drugs for cattle include the Animal Medicinal

Drug Use Clarification Act (AMDUCA, 1994) for extralabel use, the Controlled Substances Act, state pharmacy laws, and state practice acts.[12]

Drugs not approved for cattle or not approved for the production class of cattle being treated should be used following AMDUCA regulations. Medications labeled for cattle or that production class should always be considered first for treatment or control of disease.[12] If these are deemed ineffective, AMDUCA allows extralabel use of drugs under specified conditions.[14,15] The AMDUCA places constraints on veterinarians to advise extralabel usage. There must be a valid VCPR and specific circumstances before extralabel usage is allowed[14]:

- There is no approved new animal drug labeled for the intended use and that contains the same active ingredient that is in the required dosage form and concentration, except where the veterinarian finds that the approved new animal drug is clinically ineffective for its intended use.
- Before prescribing or dispensing an approved new animal or human drug for extralabel use in food animals, the veterinarian must
  ○ Make a careful diagnosis and evaluation of the conditions for which the drug is to be used
  ○ Establish a substantially extended withdrawal period before marketing of milk, meat, eggs, or other edible products supported by appropriate scientific information, if applicable
  ○ Institute procedures to assure that the identity of the treated animal or animals is carefully maintained
  ○ Take appropriate measures to assure that assigned time frames for withdrawal are met and no illegal drug residues occur in any food-producing animal subjected to extralabel treatment.

Additional requirements must be satisfied to use an approved human-label drug in an extralabel manner in food-producing animals or to use an animal drug approved only for use in animals not intended for human consumption. Specifically, the use must be accomplished in accordance with an appropriate medical rationale and the veterinarian must take appropriate measures to assure that the animal and its food product will not enter the human food supply if there is no scientific information on human food safety when the drug is used in food-producing animals.[14] Extralabel use of approved human drugs in cattle or other food-producing animals is not permitted if an animal drug approved for use in food-producing animals can be used in an extralabel manner.[14]

A good rule of thumb for cattle veterinarians is to first use drugs approved for cattle and approved for the condition treated and, if extralabel use is necessary, consider a drug approved for cattle; followed by a drug approved for other food-producing animals; and use approved human label drugs extralabel as a last resort. It is important to understand the constraints imposed by AMDUCA on extralabel usage, including the prohibition of using drugs extralabel because they are less costly or more profitable.

Veterinarians must understand regulations governing the use of compounded drugs in cattle. It is illegal to use drugs compounded from bulk ingredients in cattle[15]; however, the Food and Drug Administration (FDA) has exercised enforcement discretion when compounding from bulk ingredients for certain poison antidotes and euthanasia products, such as the poison antidotes methylene blue or sodium nitrite.[16] In these instances, the volume of production of compounded product must be limited and not on a commercial scale. Under the Food, Drug, and Cosmetic Act, a cattle drug compounded using unapproved or bulk ingredients is adulterated[17] and the marketing of cattle for food that have been treated with these drugs may be jeopardized.

The AMDUCA regulations specify that compounded preparations should be prepared from FDA-approved animal or human drugs and, whenever possible, an animal drug should be used to compound instead of a human-label drug.[12,14] Further information on compounding drugs for use in cattle can be found on the FDA Web site.[14]

Residue avoidance is of paramount importance; therefore, a written residue avoidance protocol should be developed by the feedlot veterinarian. All feedlot personnel that work in the animal health section should be regularly trained so that everyone is familiar with the residue avoidance program. When drugs are used in accordance with the label in cattle, the labeled preharvest withdrawal time should be observed before marketing. Whenever a drug is used extralabel, such as changing the dose, frequency, duration, or production class of the animal, the labeled withdrawal period does not apply. If the feedlot veterinarian prescribes a drug extralabel in an unapproved class of cattle, there is no tolerance in the edible tissues. As such, any detectable level would be a violative residue.[12,14] Therefore, it is necessary to extend the withdrawal time to avoid detectable residues in the meat. The Food Animal Residue Avoidance Databank is an excellent, responsive source for withdrawal time information when drugs are used extralabel.[17]

Accurate recordkeeping is vital for residue avoidance. The date, product used, dosage, and route of administration should be recorded, either electronically or as hard copy. Group or individual identification should also be recorded. A trained feedlot representative should carefully review withdrawal reports and sign a release for the cattle before they are shipped for slaughter.

Although AMDUCA provides for extralabel use of injectable, topical, or orally administered animal health products under specified conditions, extralabel use of feed-grade drugs is not allowed.[14] The consulting veterinarian should work closely with the nutritionist to ensure that feed-grade products are mixed in the ration at approved levels. Recently, the pharmaceutical industry voluntarily agreed to a request by the FDA to remove all production claims for feed-grade antibiotics. In addition, by December 2016, a veterinary feed directive (VFD) will be required before adding feed-grade antibiotics to cattle rations. Ionophores are excluded from this requirement. This will require close cooperation between veterinarians and nutritionists to ensure that requirements of the VFD are met. The importance of a good working relationship between feedlot veterinarians and nutritionists has been described.[18]

Several drugs are prohibited by the FDA for use in any food-producing species, even under the extralabel provisions of AMDUCA. These include chloramphenicol, clenbuterol, diethylstilbestrol, glycopeptides, nitroimidazoles, nitrofurans, and medicated feeds. Drugs with restricted extralabel use in feedlot cattle include fluoroquinolones; phenylbutazone in female dairy cattle 20 months of age or older; and extralabel dose, duration, frequency, and route of administration of cephalosporins.[17]

Understanding regulations governing drug usage in feedlot cattle, training employees, using written protocols, having a residue avoidance program in place, and regularly reviewing the program should ensure that violative drug residues are extremely rare in beef cattle from feedlots.

HANDLING PRACTICES

Improper handling can result in fear and distress in cattle[19] and the BQA concepts attempt to prevent such situations on production units. The proper handling of cattle requires the knowledge of cattle behavior and the presence of adequate handling facilities.[20] Cattle respond to the manner in which they are handled.[20] Poor handling is a welfare issue and it may have a negative effect on production in cattle. For example, Cooke[21] showed that the fear-related behavioral responses of beef cattle to human handling affect productive, reproductive, and health characteristics.

Behavioral responses of cattle to human interaction are important to observe; however, responses to other stimuli encountered during handling are equally important and objective measures of responses to both human interaction and other stimuli can be used in the assessment of animal welfare. For example, when processing cattle, objective measures can be used to determine whether handling practices are consistent with good welfare of the animals, including number of injuries, vocalization, slipping and falling in the alley, jumping and running out of the chute, electric prod use, and chute miscatches. The BQA Feedlot Assessment Tool allows producers to self-assess or to use a third party to take such measurements and, therefore, facilitate improvement of handling practices.[22]

Vocalization can be used as a simple method for detecting welfare problems.[23] Vocalization is a reliable measure of animal welfare because it is very objective, easy to tabulate, and no sophisticated equipment is required.[23] The BQA Program has set the industry standard of vocalization while processing cattle at less than 5%.[22] Percentages of animals slipping or falling in alleys, chutes, and chute exit areas can indicate welfare problems such as improper facility maintenance.[22] Also, the percentage of animals moved with an electric prod can be assessed, and a "minimum-use goal" should be set (the industry standard is 10%).[19] Chute miscatches are defined as the animal in any position other than with its head fully outside of the chute with the balance of the body within the chute or as an animal caught in the tail or back gate and not released.[22] There should be a 0% miscatch rate during processing.[22]

Industry standards have been set for electric prod use in processing barns but a standard has not been set for loading, unloading, and transport of animals. Likely, the standard would be similar to the 10% in processing barns because cattle being loaded and unloaded have similar facilities to walk through but may balk at the prospect of entering the trailer. The same can be said for driving or moving cattle to a truck, pen, or pasture. Injury rates, electric prod use, cattle speed, and the number of fatigued cattle are all important areas to measure, and can all be measured objectively, if desired. The same industry standards can be used in driving and moving cattle as in situations previously discussed.

Finally, the handling of sick and/or injured animals can be a situation in which welfare can be demonstrated very readily as excellent or severely compromised. The implementation of BQA welfare concepts are of utmost importance in such situations. Sick animals can be ambulatory or nonambulatory. They can also become nonambulatory if proper handling techniques are not used. Electric prods should be used at a minimum (less than industry standard of 10%).[22] Vocalization can also be used as a measure of welfare for handling sick or injured animals. Cattle in situations previously discussed should always be handled with care and at the pace that the animal sets. The use of best management practices, such as those outlined in the BQA Feedlot Assessment Tool, will help to facilitate improvement in handling not only sick and injured animals but all cattle.

CATTLE COMFORT

Cattle comfort should be an important consideration when considering both production and animal welfare. The importance of pen conditions, including water tank and bunk conditions, is stressed in BQA principles. All cattle should have enough pen space to get up, lie down, and move freely within their given environment. In the pens, clean water should be available at all times. Feed bunks should be clean and free of spoiled or moldy feedstuffs. The BQA Assessment tools give recommendations on monitoring and reporting the conditions of pens, water tanks, and feed bunks.[22]

Another indicator of cattle comfort is the presence of excessive mud or feces in the pens, or on and in the animals' coats. In winter conditions, if an animal's coat is wet and muddy, energy requirements for maintenance for that animal can easily double.[24] BQA concepts stress that all cattle should have a dry area in which they can lie down and rest. Cattle should also be able to get to feed and water without being required to walk through mud above their fetlock.[22] This could not only improve the welfare of the animals but also increase performance parameters.

Extreme weather conditions also have an effect on cattle comfort. The risk of heat stress for cattle is influenced by environmental factors, including air temperature, relative humidity, and wind speed; as well as animal factors, including breed, age, body condition, metabolic rate, and coat color or density.[25,26] Cattle can also be subject to stress from cold and/or wet conditions.[27] BQA guidelines give recommendations on putting management plans in place to alleviate the negative impact of increased environmental stress on cattle.

FEEDLOT HEALTH PROGRAMS ARE PART OF BEEF QUALITY ASSURANCE

Preventive medicine and therapeutic programs developed by the feedlot veterinarian address cattle's well-being. In addition, healthy cattle perform better than those that have suffered bovine respiratory disease or lameness. Within a VCPR, diagnostics, records analysis, and employee training all contribute to a successful health program. Bovine respiratory disease and diagnostic pathology are discussed in previous editions of this journal.[28,29]

CONSIDERATIONS FOR PAIN MANAGEMENT DUE TO CASTRATION AND DEHORNING

Societal concern about the treatment of animals is becoming more common, especially in food-producing animals. Although there are numerous options for effective control of pain in companion animals and horses, choices are limited for use in food-producing animals. Historically, attempts to reduce pain during common feedlot surgical procedures have been minimal. Veterinarians providing service to feedlots should provide written protocols detailing castration methods and horn management. Other surgical procedures are rarely performed on feedlot cattle.

The American Veterinary Medical Association (AVMA) and AABP have each developed guidelines or policies for castration and dehorning of cattle[30,31] AABP guidelines state that banding or surgical castration are preferred over other methods and the veterinarian should recommend the method that is in the best interest of the health and well-being of the animal within the environment in which the animal is being raised. AVMA policy states that the method used for castration should consider the animal's age, weight, skill level of the operator or technician, the environment, and the safety of the animal and people involved in the process.

Most packers will accept cattle from feedlots with horns that do not extend beyond the tips of the ears. Tipping horns of feedlot cattle should not be done merely for cosmetic reasons. Dehorning is contraindicated because of pain, the length of time to heal during the feeding period, and risk of sinus infection. A rule of thumb is to tip horns only when necessary to meet marketing requirements, and tip no more horn length than required by the packer. If horns are large, an option is to perform a cornual horn block using 2% lidocaine, which is a quick, inexpensive procedure.[32]

Options for providing systemic analgesia when castrating bulls or tipping horns is limited under commercial feedlot conditions and the use of these products is extralabel. Meloxicam, an nonsteroidal antiinflammatory drug, has been shown to reduce pain in cattle following castration and dehorning. Although there is an injectable companion animal formulation available in the United States, the cost is prohibitive. Low-cost tablets are available and bioavailability of meloxicam when administered orally is very good. At the suggested dose of 1 mg/kg, a 21-day preharvest withdrawal time is recommended. A comprehensive review of managing pain associated with castration and horn surgery has recently been published.[33,34]

Whatever the method of castration and horn management chosen, the feedlot veterinarian should ensure that employees performing the procedure are thoroughly trained on proper technique, sanitation, use of prescribed pain mitigating products, and proper aftercare.

The beef industry must continue to call for wide adoption of castration and horn management early in the calf's life, more research on new methods or techniques to eliminate pain and distress associated with surgeries in cattle, and development of effective pain-mitigating medication for cattle.

MONITORING FEED-RELATED PROBLEMS

Nearly all feedlot managers engage the services of a nutritionist. In most cases, this is an independent consulting nutritionist; however, some nutritionists are employed by a feed company at which services may or may not be tied to feed or supplement purchases. The consulting nutritionist is responsible for advising feedlot management on procurement of feed commodities, ration formulation, feed manufacturing, quality control, and delivery of feed.[18]

A good working relationship between the consulting veterinarian and consulting nutritionist is essential because health issues can compromise feeding performance, such as daily gain and feed conversion, and an overly aggressive or poorly executed feeding program can cause significant health issues. Consequently, management should encourage teamwork between all departments in the feedlot, animal health, feeding, and maintenance, to optimize health, well-being, and performance of feedlot cattle.

Veterinarians and nutritionists should routinely look for signs that suggest cattle are overly stressed by the diet. Examples include fecal consistency, acidosis or bloat syndrome, laminitis, demeanor, and variation in daily feed intake.[18] The veterinarian should notify the nutritionist when feed-related issues are discovered while performing clinical examination of animals in the feedlot or during necropsy examinations. Likewise, the nutritionist should advise the veterinarian during his or her visit when problems are spotted, such as sick cattle not pulled for treatment, unexpected increased morbidity, or hospital overcrowding. The nutritionist is in an ideal position to benchmark feeding-related issues that may compromise cattle well-being, such as the incidence of acidosis or bloat, or the prevalence of liver abscesses reported when the cattle are slaughtered.[18]

Through training of feedlot employees, providing protocols, monitoring outcomes, and teamwork, veterinarians and nutritionists can have a significant impact on performance, health and well-being of cattle in the feedlot.

MANAGEMENT OF NONAMBULATORY (DOWNER) FEEDLOT CATTLE

Downer syndrome in feedlot cattle can occur for a variety of reasons, with either sudden or gradual onset. The well-being of nonambulatory cattle can be compromised quickly if prompt action to provide supportive care is not taken. The veterinarian should provide a written protocol for the care and handling of nonambulatory cattle and provide ongoing training for management of compromised animals. It should be clear that nonambulatory cattle cannot enter the human food chain.

Pen riders should force cattle to their feet when riding pens to better evaluate the cattle for the presence of infectious disease and to quickly find cattle with compromised musculoskeletal problems because most nonambulatory cattle go down in their home feeding pen.[35] For example, cattle with a fracture may be bright, alert, and chew their cud while lying in the pen, and could easily go unnoticed if not forced to rise. The welfare of these cases is compromised if not discovered and addressed in a timely manner.

The protocol for managing nonambulatory cattle should guide the feedlot health care staff to determine whether to humanely euthanize the animal or to provide additional care. A nonambulatory animal with a good prognosis for recovery is one that is not in distress, has no severe injury, is bright and alert, continues to eat and drink, and makes frequent attempts to rise. Cattle meeting these criteria are candidates for additional care and treatment as outlined in the feedlot protocol but should be evaluated at least twice daily for evidence of improvement or deterioration.[36]

In most cases, candidates for additional care should be moved from the feeding pen to a hospital pen or barn. Personnel should be trained to humanely move nonambulatory cattle. The animal can be subjected to painful, inhumane injury if not handled properly. When moving a downed animal, it should not be dragged and should not be lifted with chains or ropes. Acceptable methods of transporting downers include a sled or rolling them into a loader bucket. Most feedlots own loaders with a bucket large enough to move cattle of any weight and size. Feedlot employees should be trained to avoid "scooping" a nonambulatory steer or heifer into the bucket because of the high risk of severe injury. Instead, the animal should be rolled into the bucket; this usually requires 2 to 3 people to safely accomplish.[37]

Nonambulatory cattle should be placed in a dry area, preferably on sand or straw bedding to reduce ischemic muscle necrosis. Ischemic muscle necrosis can occur within 6 hours after the animal goes down due to interference with the normal blood supply.[38] Selection of bedding and rolling the animal from side to side will reduce risk of muscle necrosis. Provision of shade in the heat of summer and windbreaks in the winter reduces environmental stress on the animal. Nonambulatory cattle with a favorable prognosis should be provided feed and water, and medical conditions should be treated according to the feedlot protocol.

Nonambulatory cattle with an unfavorable prognosis, such as severe injury or illness, refusal to eat or drink, or inability to sit up unaided, should be humanely euthanized within 24 to 36 hours of initial onset.[37] When severe weather conditions exist, such as a winter blizzard, it may be more humane to euthanize nonambulatory cattle sooner to avoid further distress and suffering.

A key to proper care of nonambulatory cattle is for the veterinarian and feedlot manager to foster a culture of caring. Nonambulatory cattle depend much more on human intervention than normal cattle. The feedlot is a challenging environment for these cattle; therefore, training and motivation of caretakers to consistently offer a high level of care is essential.

HUMANE EUTHANASIA

Euthanasia is one of the most important aspects of animal welfare in food animal production units and BQA concepts ensure that the procedure is done in a humane manner. Euthanasia should be implemented when an animal is experiencing a condition that has not responded to treatment and unnecessary suffering must be prevented. It is the responsibility of the persons who own or work with livestock to have the proper equipment and knowledge to conduct the procedure effectively.[39] To avoid undue pain and distress, euthanasia techniques must cause immediate loss of consciousness, followed by cardiac and respiratory arrest, and finally loss of brain function. Persons who perform this task must be proficient and have an understanding of the relevant anatomic landmarks used for humane euthanasia of cattle.[39] Protocols for the humane euthanasia of cattle are important in BQA assessments because they aid in guiding designated persons in the proper execution of the procedure. Protocols should include the persons designated to perform the humane euthanasia and the proper techniques that should be used. The method of euthanasia should also be specified. An explanation of the signs used for confirmation of death of cattle should be included. Persons who are designated to perform the task of humane euthanasia should be familiar with BQA concepts and the production unit's written protocol for humane euthanasia.

SUMMARY

The BQA program was written by beef producers and veterinarians for beef producers and veterinarians. The program has continued to evolve from its starting point of antibiotic residue avoidance to include animal handling, cattle comfort, food safety, and much more. Providing guidance to producers and veterinarians on best management practices allows the beef industry to be transparent and open about the practices employees on cattle to the beef consumer. The addition of an editor - in - the - field assessment tool provides producers guidance on implementation of BQA practices in their operation. The valid VCPR is core to the BQA program. Veterinarians are key components to helping producers implement BQA in their beef operations.

REFERENCES

1. Smith RA, Stokka GL, Radostits OM, et al. Health and production management in feedlots. In: Radostits OM, editor. Herd health – food animal production medicine. 3rd edition. Philadelphia: WB Saunders; 2001. p. 581–633.
2. Beef Cattle Institute. Animal care training. Available at: https://www.animalcaretraining.org/index.aspx. Accessed March 02, 2015.
3. Beef Quality Assurance. BQA program resources. Available at: http://www.bqa.org/resources.aspx. Accessed March 02, 2015.
4. George MH, Heinrich PE, Dexter DR, et al. Injection site lesions in carcasses produced by cattle receiving injections at branding and at weaning. J Anim Sci 1995; 73:3235–40.
5. George MH, Ames RA, Glock RG, et al. Incidence, severity, amount of tissue affected and effect on histology, chemistry and tenderness of injection site lesions in beef cuts from calves administered a control compound or one of seven chemical compounds. Final report to the National Cattlemen's Beef Association. Ft Collins (CO): Dept. of Animal Sciences, Colorado State University; 1995. p. 1–44.
6. BQA National Manual. A study of injection site lesions. p. 122–4. Available at: http://www.bqa.org/cmdocs/bqa/nationalmanual.pdf. Accessed March 02, 2015.
7. BQA National Manual. Best management practices – animal treatments and health maintenance. p. 30–2. Available at: http://www.bqa.org/cmdocs/bqa/nationalmanual.pdf. Accessed March 02, 2015.

8. Smith RA. Preharvest beef quality. In: VanOverbeke DL, editor. Handbook of beef safety and quality. Binghamton (NY): Haworth (now Taylor & Francis); 2007. p. 101–24.

9. BQA National Manual. Injection site diagrams. p. 68–71. Available at: http://www.bqa.org/cmdocs/bqa/nationalmanual.pdf. Accessed March 03, 2015.

10. AVMA. Veterinarian's oath. 2011. Available at: https://www.avma.org/KB/Policies/Pages/veterinarians-oath.aspx. Accessed February 23, 2015.

11. AABP. Establishing and maintaining the veterinarian-client-patient relationship in bovine practice. 2013. Available at: http://www.aabp.org/resources/AABP_member_Guidelines.asp. Accessed February 23, 2015.

12. AABP. Drug use guidelines for bovine practice. 2015. Available at: http://www.aabp.org/resources/aabp_guidelines/druguseguidelines_2015-4-8-1.pdf

13. Sundlof SF. Legal control of veterinary drugs. In: Adams HR, editor. Veterinary pharmacology, and therapeutics. 8th edition. Ames (IA): Iowa State University Press; 2001. p. 1149–56.

14. U.S. Food and Drug Administration. Animal Medicinal Drug Use Clarification Act. 1994. Available at: http://www.fda.gov/AnimalVeterinary/GuidanceComplianceEnforcement/ActsRulesRegulations/ucm085377.htm#Food-Producing_Animals. Accessed February 19, 2015.

15. U.S. Government Printing Office. Electronic Code of Federal Regulations: 21CFR530.13. Extra-label use from compounding of approved new animal and approved human drugs. 2015. Available at: http://www.ecfr.gov/cgi-bin/text-idx?SID=054808d261de27898e02fb175b7c9ff9&node=21:6.0.1.1.16&rgn=div5#21:6.0.1.1.16.2.1.4. Accessed February 28, 2015.

16. U.S. Food and Drug Administration. Inspections, compliance and criminal investigations. CPG Sec 608.400. Compounding of drugs for use in animals. 2014. Available at: http://www.fda.gov/iceci/compliancemanuals/compliancepolicyguidancemanual/ucm074656.htm. Accessed February 27, 2015.

17. Food Animal Residue Avoidance Databank. Available at: http://www.farad.org/eldu/prohibit.asp. Accessed March 03, 2015.

18. Smith RA, Hollis LC. Interaction between consulting veterinarians and nutritionists in the feedlot. Vet Clin North Am Food Anim Pract 2007;23:171–5.

19. Grandin T. Recommended animal handling guidelines and audit guide: a systematic approach to animal welfare. American Meat Institution Foundation; 2010. Available at: http://www.grandin.com/meat.institute.menu.html.

20. Bicudo JR, Burris R, Laurent K, et al. Handling beef cattle. University of Kentucky College of Agriculture, Food, and Environment 2003. Available at: http://www2.ca.uky.edu/agc/pubs/id/id108/03.pdf.

21. Cooke RF. Bill E. Kunkle interdisciplinary beef symposium: temperament and acclimation to human handling influence growth, health, and reproductive responses in Bos taurus and Bos indicus cattle. J Anim Sci 2014;92:5325–33.

22. Beef Quality Assurance Feedlot Assessment. 2010. Available at: www.bqa.org/assessments. Accessed March 10, 2015.

23. Grandin T. The feasibility of using vocalization scoring as an indicator of poor welfare during cattle slaughter. Appl Anim Behav Sci 1998;56:121–8.

24. Mader TL. Mud effects on feedlot cattle. Nebraska Beef Cattle Report 2011;81–3.

25. Gaughan JB, Mader TL, Holt SM, et al. Assessing the heat tolerance of 17 beef cattle genotypes. Int J Biometeorol 2010;54:617–27.

26. Mader TL, Davis MS, Brown-Brandl T. Environmental factors influencing heat stress in feedlot cattle. J Anim Sci 2006;84:712–9.

27. Mader TL. Bill E. Kunkle Interdisciplinary Beef Symposium: animal welfare concerns for cattle exposed to adverse environmental conditions. J Anim Sci 2014;92:5319–24.
28. Cooper VL, Broderson BW. Bovine respiratory disease. Vet Clin North Am Food Anim Pract 2010;26:409–16.
29. Cooper VL. Diagnostic pathology. Vet Clin North Am Food Anim Pract 2012;28:xi.
30. American Association of Bovine Practitioners. Castration and dehorning guidelines. 2014. Available at: http://www.aabp.org/resources/aabp_guidelines/castration_and_dehorning_guidelines_app3.2014_03.17.2014.pdf. Accessed March 07, 2015.
31. American Veterinary Medical Association. Castration and dehorning of cattle. 2014. Available at: https://www.avma.org/KB/Policies/Pages/Castration-and-Dehorning-of-Cattle.aspx. Accessed March 07, 2015.
32. Noordsy JL, Ames NK. Local and regional anesthesia. In: Food animal surgery. 4th edition. Yardley (PA): Veterinary Learning Systems; 2006. p. 21–42.
33. Coetzee JF. Assessment and management of pain associated with castration in cattle. Vet Clin North Am Food Anim Pract 2013;29:76–101.
34. Stock ML, Baldridge SL, Griffin DD, et al. Bovine dehorning: assessing pain and providing analgesic management. Vet Clin North Am Food Anim Pract 2013;29:103–33.
35. Portillo TA. Pen riding and evaluation of cattle in pens to identify compromised individuals. Proceedings of the 47th Annual Conference of the American Association of Bovine Practitioners, vol. 47. Stillwater (OK): VM Publishing; 2014. p. 5–8.
36. AABP. AABP position statement on the care of non-ambulatory and injured ambulatory cattle. 2013. Available at: http://www.aabp.org/resources/aabp_position_statements/AABP_Non-ambulatory_Cattle-06.2013.pdf. Accessed February 28, 2015.
37. BQA Cattle Care and Handling Guidelines. Non-ambulatory (downer) cattle: p. 15. Available at: http://www.bqa.org/CMDocs/bqa/CCHG2015_Final.pdf. Accessed March 01, 2015.
38. Shearer J, van Amstel SR. Upper leg lameness. In: Manual for treatment and control of lameness in cattle. Ames (IA): Blackwell; 2006. p. 147–64.
39. BQA Cattle Care and Handling Guidelines. Humane euthanasia: p. 16. Available at: http://www.bqa.org/CMDocs/bqa/CCHG2015_Final.pdf. Accessed March 15, 2015.

Nutrition of Newly Received Feedlot Cattle

Chris Reinhardt, PhD[a],*, Daniel U. Thomson, DVM, PhD[b]

KEYWORDS

- Feedlot • Stress • Calves • Diet • Nutrition • Water • Rumen

KEY POINTS

- The stress of transition from pasture to the feedlot environment creates unique and variable nutritional challenges.
- The more time that calves do not have access to good-quality feed and water in the course of this transition process, the greater the level of challenge and the greater the urgency to reestablish some normalcy to the rumen environment.
- The factors that are used to assign a risk category for the likelihood of developing bovine respiratory disease include time in transit from their origin, which is likely to be highly correlated with the amount of time away from quality feed and water.
- A high risk of developing respiratory disease is likely to correlate well with the animals' suppressed appetite immediately after arrival.

HIGH-RISK CALVES
Water

High-risk calves are subjected to various degrees of physiologic and psychological stress, physical exhaustion, immune system suppression, viral and bacterial respiratory pathogen challenge, and water and feed deprivation. Therefore, there are 3 primary needs that must be addressed soon after arrival: water, feed, and rest.

Any discussion of either human or animal nutrition must begin with a discussion of water. Cattle under no abnormal stress typically drink 3 times their normal dry matter intake (DMI) in water; during heat stress conditions, cattle may increase that amount to 5 times their feed intake to compensate for water lost through extensive evaporative cooling from the lungs and the surface of the skin. Arias and Mader[1] suggest that during extremely warm weather daily water consumption can more than double (**Fig. 1**).

The authors have nothing to disclose.
[a] Department of Animal Sciences and Industry, Kansas State University, 136 Call Hall, Manhattan, KS 66506-1600, USA; [b] Diagnostic Medicine and Pathobiology, Kansas State University, 1-D Trotter Hall, Manhattan, KS 66506-1600, USA
* Corresponding author.
E-mail address: cdr3@ksu.edu

Vet Clin Food Anim 31 (2015) 283–294
http://dx.doi.org/10.1016/j.cvfa.2015.03.010
0749-0720/15/$ – see front matter Published by Elsevier Inc.

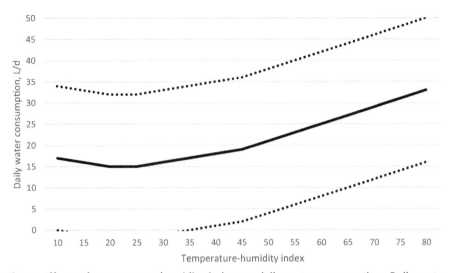

Fig. 1. Effects of temperature humidity index on daily water consumption. Daily water intake = $22.224 - 0.651x + 0.0175x^2 - 8.7e{-}5x^3$; Adj. $R^2 = 0.61$. Dotted lines indicate the 95% confidence interval. (*Data from* Arias RA, Mader TL. Environmental factors affecting daily water intake on cattle finished in feedlots. J Anim Sci 2011;89:245–51.)

During warm weather, extra water sources may need to be made available, such as large, metal, portable tanks. Water should be clean, cool, and fresh. For cattle that have never used an automatic water trough, the floats may need to be fixed open. The sound of the flowing water may help attract the calves, and this also prevents calves from being spooked by the sound of a sudden rush of water filling the emptying trough while calves are drinking. Water tanks may be placed on the perimeter of the pen to provide additional drinking space for calves. Calves often walk the perimeter of their new pen, and placing tanks in their path helps make them aware of the water source. Other critical elements that increase the need for additional water sources include whether calves have been off feed and water for an extended period, whether calves have never used an automatic water trough, whether water pressure in the feed yard cannot accommodate a high volume of water demand over a short time, and whether some calves are extremely timid and will not compete with the group for access to water.

The rumen and its microbial populations function best when the animal's own physiology is able to closely regulate the rumen environment within the range of normalcy. Under ideal circumstances, the animal consumes forage and chews the forage to reduce the particle size and provide access for microbes. The forage is buffered by saliva and then swallowed; that forage is fermented for a time, is regurgitated, rechewed, rebuffered, and reswallowed. The volatile fatty acids produced from forage fermentation are absorbed through the rumen wall or pass out with the liquid phase; acids produced through normal fermentation are buffered by saliva. After the physical rumen fill is sufficiently reduced through digestion and passage out of the rumen, the animal grazes for additional forage substrate. This repeated cycle of consumption, buffering, breakdown, and removal of fermentation end products and undigested forage results in a fairly controlled ruminal pH and environment, optimizing fermentation.

Hay

- Hay should be provided free choice, in the bunk, immediately on arrival.
- Hay feeding can be continued on the day after arrival in addition to the starter diet. Subsequently, hay feeding should only be continued if calves refuse to eat the starter diet.

If calves have been off feed and water for a protracted period, they will be both thirsty and hungry. If they are not completely exhausted, some or all of the calves will seek out feed and water; have both readily available before calves arrive. For calves that may not understand where feed can be accessed, fresh, clean, long-stemmed, high-quality hay should be placed in the feed bunk. To attract timid calves, some of this hay can be spread behind the bunk inside the pen on the bunk pad. Good-quality, digestible hay with long particle length is a good source of nutrients for rumen microbes but also stimulates eating, chewing, and salivary buffer production by the calves. Lofgreen and colleagues[2] showed that calves that had access to free-choice hay had reduced death loss and greater average daily gain (ADG) than those that only received the complete diet (**Table 1**).

Healthy calves have the ability to consume 3% or more of their body weight as dry matter of good-quality hay. However, the goal is not to fill calves with hay; if calves are aggressive and have recovered from the transition stress, it is preferred to get them quickly transitioned onto a fully fortified complete receiving diet. For this reason, hay should be limited to 1.5% of body weight as dry matter, and should only be continued for calves that refuse to consume an adequate quantity of the receiving diet. Lofgreen and colleagues[3] reported that calves fed a 75% concentrate receiving diet with access to hay had greater ADG during the first week postarrival, but allowing unlimited access to hay during the second, third, and fourth weeks after arrival resulted in numerically poorer performance (**Table 2**).

For extremely timid animals that are reluctant to approach the front of the pen, a bale ring can be placed at the center of the pen to allow these timid calves to regain some of their lost fill and provide them with energy. However, this works contrary to the goal of teaching calves to come to the bunk, but it may be essential to provide feed access for extremely stressed calves. If a bale ring is used, this should be practiced only for 1 to 2 days.

On the day of arrival, 1% to 1.5% of body weight of hay should be placed loose and long-stemmed in the bunk and then top dressed with 0.25% to 0.5% of body weight of a complete, mixed, receiving diet. This diet commonly contains processed grain,

Table 1		
Effects of free-choice hay on death loss in feedlot calves during the first 56 days after arrival		
Item	**No Hay**	**Free-choice Alfalfa Hay**
Number of calves	258	256
Number of calves that died	13[a]	7[a]
Days treated	142[a]	121[a]
Number of calves retreated	24[a]	16[a]
ADG (g)	458[a]	816[a]
Feed/gain ratio	8.67[a]	5.52[a]

[a] Means within a row without common superscripts differ.

Data from Lofgreen GP, Stinocher IH, Kiesling HE. Effects of dietary energy, free choice alfalfa hay and mass medication on calves subjected to marketing and shipping stresses. J Anim Sci 1980;50:590–6.

Table 2
Effects of allowing free-choice access to hay on ADG during the first, second, third, and fourth weeks postarrival

	Millet Hay Alone	Alfalfa Hay Alone	75% Concentrate Diet With No Hay	With Hay
Week 1	2.51[a]	2.27[a]	2.75[a]	4.16[a]
Week 2	0.92[a]	1.74[a]	3.08[a]	2.86[a]
Week 3	0.33[a]	1.30[a]	2.99[a]	2.62[a]
Week 4	1.10[a]	1.39[a]	2.13[a]	1.61[a]

[a] Means within a row without common superscripts differ.
Data from Lofgreen GP, Stinocher IH, Kiesling HE. Effects of dietary energy, free choice alfalfa hay and mass medication on calves subjected to marketing and shipping stresses. J Anim Sci 1980;50:590–6.

processed forage, a complete balanced supplement, and any feed grade medications recommended. If all the hay is consumed by the second day, 0.5% of body weight of hay can be fed.

Intake Issues

- Healthy, nonstressed calves have the potential to consume 3% of body weight of a receiving diet.
- Highly stressed calves often consume 1.5% of body weight or less, on a dry matter basis, during the first 2 weeks postarrival.

Tissues and organs of cattle do not function on ratios, such as percentages or parts per million (ppm). Instead, the animals' tissues have needs for specific quantities (eg, milligrams, grams, pounds, and kilograms) of all essential nutrients. The specific levels of nutrients required vary based on animal size and weight, sex, physiologic age, and stage of production. However, because high-risk calves typically consume less feed per unit of body weight than a similar calf under no transitional stress, the ratio of these essential nutrients must be increased in the diet to a degree; the degree of increase is a point of much debate.

Hutcheson and Cole[4] showed that high-risk calves, following an extended time in transit, require several weeks before achieving normal consumption levels (**Table 3**). Chirase and colleagues[5] showed that calves experimentally infected with bovine herpes virus-1 (BHV-1) had a 30% to 75% reduction in dry matter intake compared with prechallenge levels (**Fig. 2**). Hutcheson and Cole[4] reported that on day 7 postarrival only 83% of morbid calves had eaten at some point during the first 7 days after arrival, whereas 95% of healthy calves had eaten; only 43% to 70% of morbid calves ate feed on any given day during days 2 to 7 postarrival, whereas 62% to 88% of healthy calves were eating each day (**Table 4**).

Table 3
Expected dry matter intake of newly received, high-risk feedlot calves

Time After Arrival	Dry Matter Intake (% of Body Weight)
Day 1–7	0.5–1.5
Day 8–14	1.5–2.5
Day 14–28	2.5–3.5

Data from Hutcheson DP, Cole NA. Management of transit-stress syndrome in cattle: nutritional and environmental effects. J Anim Sci 1986;62:555–60.

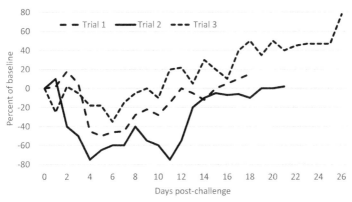

Fig. 2. Effect of BHV-1 challenge on dry matter intake in calves. (*Data from* Chirase NK, Hutcheson DP, Thompson GB. Feed intake, rectal temperature, and serum mineral concentrations of feedlot cattle fed zinc oxide or zinc methionine and challenged with infectious bovine rhinotracheitis virus. J Anim Sci 1991;69:4137–45.)

A feed yard that only receives a single load of high-risk calves can use dry matter intake on any given day to reformulate the amount of nutrient increase required. However, because most feed yards receive many loads of these calves, often in rapid succession, and because each load and pen has a unique level of intake, some compromise must be made as to the appropriate level of nutrient fortification of the receiving diet. Even healthy calves do not consume up to their full potential for several weeks after transport stress (**Table 5**), but morbid calves lag behind their healthy counterparts even out to 56 days on feed.

Concentrate

- Forage content of the receiving and starting diet should be maintained at 40% on a dry matter basis, with the remainder made up of grain, protein, minerals, and vitamins.
- The forage used should be a good-quality grass hay or alfalfa-grass hay mix.
- Silage can be used but should be limited to less than 30% of diet dry matter.

Table 4
Percentage of calves consuming feed

Day	Percentage Eating on that Day Healthy	Morbid	Cumulative Percentage Having Eaten at Some Point During the Previous Days Healthy	Morbid
1	39	27	39	27
2	62	43	66	47
3	82	59	85	67
4	83	62	89	76
5	86	67	90	80
6	89	67	95	82
7	88	70	95	83

Data from Hutcheson DP, Cole NA. Management of transit-stress syndrome in cattle: nutritional and environmental effects. J Anim Sci 1986;62:555–60.

Table 5
Dry matter intake (percentage of body weight) of healthy and morbid calves during the first 56 days postarrival at the feedlot

	Dry Matter Intake (% of Body Weight)	
Time	Healthy	Morbid
Day 1–7	1.55	0.90
Day 1–28	2.71	1.84
Day 1–56	3.03	2.68

Data from Hutcheson DP, Cole NA. Management of transit-stress syndrome in cattle: nutritional and environmental effects. J Anim Sci 1986;62:555–60.

Although healthy calves consuming a forage diet can compensate for the decrease in dietary energy concentration by increasing voluntary intake, stressed and depressed calves do not. The reverse is true: Fluharty and Loerch[6] found that voluntary dry matter intake of stressed calves increased with increasing concentrate percentage. Lofgreen[7] reported that when highly stressed calves were permitted to select their diet, they chose a diet that averaged 72% concentrate and 28% forage. However, calves consuming high-concentrate diets may experience additional stress caused by acidosis, resulting in greater morbidity and mortality.[8]

Protein

- Protein concentration should be targeted at 14% to 16% of diet dry matter with most of the supplemental crude protein being supplied by high-quality plant sources.
- Urea should be limited to no more than 0.35% of diet dry matter.

The protein concentration should be increased in the receiving diet because of low intake but also because active challenges to immune function elicit a catabolic response, resulting in tissue protein mobilization. Boyles and colleagues[9] showed that nitrogen balance shifted away from tissue stores following BHV-1 challenge (**Fig. 3**). Nitrogen moving toward tissue deposition decreases by 49%; nitrogen being released from tissue increases by 43%, and nitrogen excretion increases by 79%, indicating a catabolic state. In addition, Cole and colleagues[10] reported 49% and 43% increases in urinary and fecal nitrogen excretion immediately following 9-hour transport. Feeding an increased level of protein (14%–16% crude protein) in the

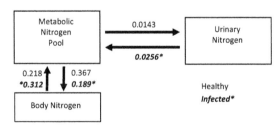

Fig. 3. Effects of BHV-1 challenge on nitrogen balance. (*Adapted from* Boyles DW, Richardson CR, Cobb CS, et al. Influence of protein status on the severity of the hypermetabolic response of calves with infectious bovine rhinotracheitis virus. Texas Tech University Animal Science Report 1989;T-5-263:15.)

receiving diet may alleviate a portion of the hypercatabolism incurred during stress,[9] resulting in more rapid recovery of weight lost during transport. However, there is evidence that feeding even greater levels of crude protein may exacerbate stress and further contribute to morbidity and mortality.[11]

Potassium

Potassium should be formulated at 1.2% to 1.4% of diet dry matter in the receiving diet.

Potassium is a critical electrolyte that is lost in response to dehydration; replenishing the potassium status is essential for normal immune and metabolic functions. Hutcheson and colleagues[12] reported that feeding an increased level of potassium in the receiving diet of high-risk calves resulted in numerical reductions in death loss and ADG postarrival (**Table 6**).

Wet Ingredients

Wet ingredients, such as liquid molasses and wet corn milling by-products, may improve the condition of the diet and reduce fines and sorting of the diet in the bunk, but total moisture content of the receiving diet should not exceed 30%.

Corn silage can be used to a limited extent; however, high-risk calves may have an aversion to the odor of corn silage and therefore it should be included with caution. If

Table 6
Effects of increased potassium intake on postshipping performance

Trial 1	Potassium Level 0.9%		Potassium Level 1.4%	
Number of animals	53		54	
Morbidity (n)	12		7	
Mortality (n)	2		0	
ADG (kg/d), 28 d				
55% concentrate diet preshipment	1.41[a]		1.48[a]	
Hay preshipment	1.22[a]		1.40[a]	

Trial 2	Potassium Level 0.7%	Potassium Level 1.3%	Potassium Level 2.2%	Potassium Level 3.1%
Number of animals	40	40	40	40
Morbidity (n)	20	21	19	21
Mortality (n)	6	1	1	5
ADG (kg/d)				
Hay preshipment				
28 d	0.56	0.73	0.71	0.69
49 d	0.56[a]	0.63[a]	0.66[a]	0.62[a]
55% concentrate diet preshipment				
28 d	0.69	0.66	0.63	0.70
49 d	0.63[a]	0.63[a]	0.56[a]	0.65[a]

[a] Means within a row without common superscripts differ ($P<.05$).

Data from Hutcheson DP, Cole NA, McLaren JB. Effects of pretransit diets and post-transit potassium levels for feeder calves. J Anim Sci 1984;58:700–8.

corn silage is used in the receiving diet its inclusion should be limited to no greater than 30% of the diet dry matter.[6]

Trace Minerals

- Copper should be formulated at 10 to 15 ppm.
- Zinc should be formulated at 75 to 100 ppm.[13]

Copper and zinc are mobilized from the body stores during stress and immune challenge. Serum zinc levels decrease in the days following viral infection, but return to normal following supplementation (**Table 7**).[5] Calves that were determined to be morbid after arrival had similar serum zinc levels to their healthy counterparts but had depressed serum zinc levels in the days following arrival (**Table 8**).[14] However, the difference diminishes with time after supplementation.

Serum copper concentration does not decrease during disease as does serum zinc (see **Table 8**), but instead increases in both morbid and healthy calves in response to the stress of the transition process (**Table 9**).[14] Most serum copper is bound to ceruloplasmin, levels of which increase during stress.[15] Excretion of both copper and zinc through the urine increases in response to viral infection (**Fig. 4**),[14] emphasizing that these resources have been lost and need to be replenished through the diet.

Vitamins

Vitamin A should be supplemented at a rate of 3960 to 5940 IU/kg (1800–2700 IU/lb) of dry matter in the receiving diet.[13]

Vitamin A is essential for maintenance of epithelial cell integrity[16] and contributes to improved humoral immune function.[17] Vitamin A, being a fat-soluble vitamin, is typically in high supply in liver stores following extended grazing of green forages. However, if calves have been grazing in areas of little rainfall or have been foraging on dormant winter pasture, vitamin A stores may be depleted. Vitamin A content of feeds, particularly forages, can be highly variable; therefore, supplementation is advantageous.

Vitamin E should be supplemented at a rate of 101 IU/kg (46 IU/lb) of dry matter in the receiving diet.[13]

Vitamin E is associated with selenium in acting as an antioxidant,[18] but also contributes to enhanced humoral immune response.[19] Secrist and colleagues[20] reviewed 5 studies that evaluated the effects of providing an additional 400 to 1600 IU of vitamin E daily to transport-stressed calves after arrival at the feedlot and reported numerical improvements in ADG, feed-to-gain ratio (F/G), and morbidity (**Table 10**). The stress of weaning, commingling, transport, and handling results in reductions in circulating vitamin E levels, but supplementation normalizes circulating levels of vitamin E.[21]

Table 7					
Serum zinc concentrations (ppm) in calves experimentally infected with BHV-1					
	Day 0	Day 4	Day 7	Day 11	Day 28
Trial 1	1.40[a]	1.05[a]	—	0.91[a]	—
Trial 2	1.88[a]	—	1.22[a]	—	1.57[a]

[a] Means within a row without a common superscript differ (P<.05).

Data from Chirase NK, Hutcheson DP, Thompson GB. Feed intake, rectal temperature, and serum mineral concentrations of feedlot cattle fed zinc oxide or zinc methionine and challenged with infectious bovine rhinotracheitis virus. J Anim Sci 1991;69:4137–45.

Table 8
Serum zinc concentrations in healthy and morbid calves after feedlot arrival

	Serum Zinc (ppm)		Serum Copper (ppm)	
Days Postarrival	Healthy	Morbid	Healthy	Morbid
0	0.70	0.68	1.02	1.04
7	0.65[a]	0.45[a]	1.04	1.06
8	0.65[a]	0.48[a]	1.01	1.04
9	0.77[a]	0.48[a]	1.00[a]	1.10[a]
10	0.76	0.59	1.18	1.18

[a] Means within a row without a common superscript differ ($P<.05$).
Data from Orr CL, Hutcheson DP, Grainger RB, et al. Serum copper, zinc, calcium and phosphorus concentrations of calves stressed by bovine respiratory disease and infectious bovine rhinotracheitis. J Anim Sci 1990;68:2893–900.

Step-up Program

For the first 45 days after arrival, the greatest concern regarding the management of highly stressed calves is prevention and treatment of respiratory disease. Premature urgency to move these calves to a high-grain diet may create acidosis challenges, which may either mask respiratory disease diagnosis or exacerbate the disease. For this reason there is value in providing extra time during the first 45 days for adaptation to the step-up diets. For calves with prolonged depression of intake, there may be value in providing the starter diet for an extended period and even continuing to allow access to hay.

- Deliver 0.25% to 0.5%of the average body weight, of the receiving diet on a dry matter basis, per animal in the receiving pen on the day of arrival.
- If the calves readily consume this amount, increase the amount of diet by 0.5%of body weight daily or every second day.
- Target consumption on the starter diet is 2.5% to 3.0% of body weight before advancing onto the next diet.

Continue feeding hay in the bunk in addition to the receiving diet until calves are consuming the receiving diet consistently; ideally calves will be eating 1.5% of body

Table 9
Serum zinc concentrations in healthy and morbid calves before transport and after feedlot arrival

	Serum Zinc (ppm)		Serum Copper (ppm)	
Sampling Time	Healthy	Morbid	Healthy	Morbid
Farm of origin	1.66[a]	1.60[a]	1.03[a]	0.98[a]
Auction barn	1.53[a]	1.53[a]	1.17[a]	1.15[a]
Peak morbidity	0.97[a,b]	0.69[a,b]	1.25[a]	1.30[a]
Day 28	0.95[a]	0.93[a]	1.15[a,b]	1.27[a,b]
Day 52	1.31[a,b]	1.01[a,b]	1.19[a,b]	1.38[a,b]

[a] Means within a column without a common superscript differ.
[b] Means within a row without a common superscript differ ($P<.05$).
Data from Orr CL, Hutcheson DP, Grainger RB, et al. Serum copper, zinc, calcium and phosphorus concentrations of calves stressed by bovine respiratory disease and infectious bovine rhinotracheitis. J Anim Sci 1990;68:2893–900.

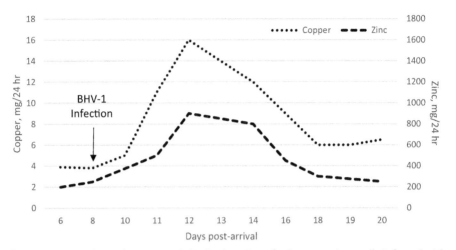

Fig. 4. Concentrations of copper and zinc in the urine of calves experimentally infected with BHV-1. (*Data from* Orr CL, Hutcheson DP, Grainger RB, et al. Serum copper, zinc, calcium and phosphorus concentrations of calves stressed by bovine respiratory disease and infectious bovine rhinotracheitis. J Anim Sci 1990;68:2893–900.)

weight by the end of the first week. Achieving consistent consumption may take only a few days or it may take more than a week, depending on the stress and disease challenge in each group of calves.

After day 45, most groups of calves will be consuming on a more consistent basis and respiratory disease, although not eliminated, will typically be declining. The cattle can be managed and stepped up conventionally from this point forward.

YEARLINGS

With respect to this article, this group may include anything from long yearlings that have been backgrounded for a season and subsequently grazed for another season, resulting in cattle with a large capacity to consume feed to weaned calves that have been backgrounded for as little as 90 days on a moderate-quality diet. The factors that the different types of cattle in this category have in common is that they are (1) not likely to be highly stressed, (2) are not at high risk to develop bovine respiratory disease, and (3) are likely to take to the bunk and to the diet readily.

Although much of the previous discussion of highly stressed calves centers on the need to (1) attract calves to the bunk, and (2) accommodate for depressed intake,

Table 10			
Effects of supplemental vitamin E for transport-stressed calves after feedlot arrival			
	No Vitamin E Added	**Vitamin E Added**	**P Value**
ADG (kg/d)	0.80	0.92	.14
DMI (kg/d)	7.48	7.49	.86
F/G ratio	12.42	9.00	.10
Morbidity (%)	55.1	47.9	.14

Data from Secrist DS, Owens FN, Gill DR. Effects of vitamin E on performance of feedlot cattle: a review. Prof Anim Sci 1997;13:47–54.

yearlings have no such needs. The high intakes of yearlings often encourage the feedlot personnel to step the cattle onto a high-grain diet too rapidly, with disastrous outcomes.

Water

All the aforementioned issues about water capacity and linear access space may be equally true for this group. If the yearlings have been without access to feed and water for an extended period, especially if cattle arrive during warm weather, it is best to provide abundant access to water.

Hay

Although the risk of respiratory disease is not as great, yearling cattle that have not had access to feed and water may be aggressive eaters. For this reason, there may be value in providing access to hay to provide both nutrients and fill. The amount of hay provided can be limited to 0.5% of body weight dry matter.

Diet

A quality starter or receiving diet works effectively for both highly stressed calves and for yearlings. The primary difference is that the yearlings, if all cattle are eating, can often be moved off the starter diet within 2 to 3 days.

Yearlings that have been on a moderate plane of energy immediately before delivery to the feed yard can be started directly on a middle step-up diet. However, if the time in transit was sufficient to create aggressive bunk behavior, there is still value in either initiating with the starter diet or providing hay on arrival.

If the feed yard does not receive any high-risk calves, the levels of protein, potassium, vitamins, and trace minerals in the starter diet can be formulated more in line with those used in the finishing diet.

In contrast with the low-intake challenge provided by highly stressed calves, yearling cattle are often aggressive eaters and eat large meals early in the step-up phase. When transitioning yearling cattle to increasingly greater concentrations of grain, avoid moving cattle up to the next diet when cattle are aggressive; instead, ensure that cattle are satisfied, or else provide the lower step diet for the first feeding of the day and then move to the higher step for subsequent feedings.

REFERENCES

1. Arias RA, Mader TL. Environmental factors affecting daily water intake on cattle finished in feedlots. J Anim Sci 2011;89:245–51.
2. Lofgreen GP, Stinocher IH, Kiesling HE. Effects of dietary energy, free choice alfalfa hay and mass medication on calves subjected to marketing and shipping stresses. J Anim Sci 1980;50:590–6.
3. Lofgreen GP, El tayeb AE, Kiesling HE. Millet and alfalfa hays alone and in combination with high-energy diet for receiving stressed calves. J Anim Sci 1981;52: 959–68.
4. Hutcheson DP, Cole NA. Management of transit-stress syndrome in cattle: nutritional and environmental effects. J Anim Sci 1986;62:555–60.
5. Chirase NK, Hutcheson DP, Thompson GB. Feed intake, rectal temperature, and serum mineral concentrations of feedlot cattle fed zinc oxide or zinc methionine and challenged with infectious bovine rhinotracheitis virus. J Anim Sci 1991;69: 4137–45.

6. Fluharty FL, Loerch SC. Effects of dietary energy source and level on performance of newly arrived feedlot calves. J Anim Sci 1996;74:504–13.
7. Lofgreen GP. Nutrition and management of stressed beef calves. Vet Clin North Am Large Anim Pract 1983;5:87–101.
8. Lofgreen GP, Dunbar JR, Addis DG, et al. Energy level in starting rations for calves subjected to marketing and shipping stress. J Anim Sci 1975;41:1256–65.
9. Boyles DW, Richardson CR, Cobb CS, et al. Influence of protein status on the severity of the hypermetabolic response of calves with infectious bovine rhinotracheitis virus. Texas Tech University Animal Science Report 1989;T-5-263:14–5.
10. Cole NA, Phillips WA, Hutcheson DP. The effect of pre-fast diet and transport on nitrogen metabolism of calves. J Anim Sci 1986;62:1719–31.
11. Galyean ML, Perino LJ, Duff GC. Interaction of cattle health/immunity and nutrition. J Anim Sci 1999;77:1120–34.
12. Hutcheson DP, Cole NA, McLaren JB. Effects of pretransit diets and post-transit potassium levels for feeder calves. J Anim Sci 1984;58:700–8.
13. National Research Council (NRC). Nutrient requirements of beef cattle. 7th revised edition. Washington, DC: National Academy Press; 1996.
14. Orr CL, Hutcheson DP, Grainger RB, et al. Serum copper, zinc, calcium and phosphorus concentrations of calves stressed by bovine respiratory disease and infectious bovine rhinotracheitis. J Anim Sci 1990;68:2893–900.
15. Qiu X, Arthington JD, Riley DG, et al. Genetic effects on acute phase protein response to the stresses of weaning and transportation in beef calves. J Anim Sci 2007;85:2367–74.
16. Scott ML, Nesheim MC, Young RJ. Nutrition of the chicken. Ithaca (NY): Scotland associates; 1982.
17. Panda B, Combs GF. Impaired antibody production in chicks fed diets low in vitamin A, pantothenic acid or riboflavin. Proc Soc Exp Biol Med 1963;113:530.
18. Latshaw JD. Nutrition - mechanisms of immunosuppression. Vet Immunol Immunopathol 1991;30:111–20.
19. Marsh JA, Dietert RR, Combs GF Jr. Influence of dietary selenium and vitamin E on the humoral immune response of the chick. Proc Soc Exp Biol Med 1981;166:228–36.
20. Secrist DS, Owens FN, Gill DR. Effects of vitamin E on performance of feedlot cattle: a review. Prof Anim Sci 1997;13:47–54.
21. Sconberg S, Nockels CF, Bennett BW, et al. Effects of shipping, handling, adrenocorticotrophic hormone, and epinephrine on α-tocopherol content of bovine blood. Am J Vet Res 1993;54:1287.

Indoor Confined Feedlots

Daniel L. Grooms, DVM, PhD[a],*, Lee Anne K. Kroll, DVM, MS[b]

KEYWORDS

- Confined feedlots • Tail necrosis • Feedlot lameness

KEY POINTS

- Indoor confined feedlots offer advantages that make them desirable in northern climates where high rainfall and snowfall occur.
- These facilities increase the risk of certain health risks, including lameness and tail injuries.
- Closed confinement can also facilitate the rapid spread of infectious disease.
- Veterinarians can help to manage these health risks by implementing management practices to reduce their occurrence.

An indoor confined feedlot (ICF) is defined as a feedlot housing system in which cattle are housed in an enclosed, under-roof facility (**Fig. 1**). These feedlots are most commonly ventilated naturally through open sides and ridge vents. Flooring can range from slatted concrete floors to solid concrete or dirt floors. An example of a slatted floor ICF is shown in **Fig. 2**. Recommended stocking density per animal for ICFs ranges from 1.1 to 2.3 m^2 (12–25 ft^2), depending on flooring type.[1] In comparison, the recommended stocking density per animal for an open dirt lot typical of western US feedlots is 45.7 to 182.8 m^2 (150–600 ft^2) depending on the design.[1] Although located throughout the United States, ICFs are most common in northern climates and especially those areas with heavy rainfall and snowfall. As an example, ICFs are commonly found in the Great Lakes region of North America.

In climatic conditions common in the Great Lakes Region of the United States, important advantages of ICFs, when compared with outdoor lots, are efficient growth and feed conversion.[2] As an example, in a study comparing similar cattle fed in a slatted floor ICF and open lots during winter months in Michigan, cattle fed in the ICF had better average daily gain (1.4 kg/d vs 1.3 kg/d [3.09 lb/d vs 2.95 lb/d]) and feed to gain ratio (7.5 vs 8.3).[3] Other studies have found similar improvements in performance in ICFs, especially in winter months.[4,5] ICFs also have the advantage

The authors have nothing to disclose.
[a] Department of Large Animal Clinical Sciences, Michigan State University, 736 Wilson Road, East Lansing, MI 48824, USA; [b] Arenec Bay Veterinary Services, 4366 M 61, Standish, MI 48658, USA
* Corresponding author.
E-mail address: grooms@cvm.msu.edu

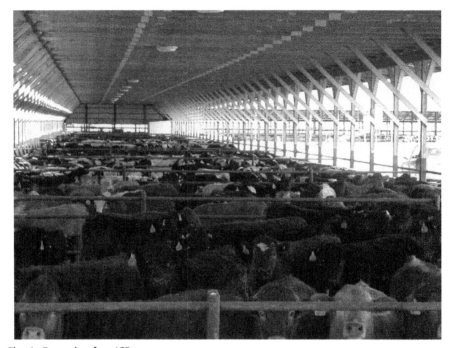

Fig. 1. Example of an ICF.

of improved ability to control manure runoff. This factor is particularly important in areas, such as the Great Lakes region, where protection of surface water resources is a top priority. From a manure quality perspective, nitrogen loss is also reduced, especially in slatted floor ICFs with associated underground pits.[6] Manure accumulation on hides is generally less, especially when housed on concrete slats. This factor is beneficial both from an economic and a food safety perspective, because excess manure tag can reduce payouts to producers and become a risk for carcass contamination during slaughter.

In contrast, animal health detriments of ICFs, and more specifically of slatted floor ICFs, include increased incidence of lameness,[7–9] increased risk for disease spread through close confinement, and increased incidence of tail tip injuries.[10–14] These detriments are described in more detail in the following sections.

TAIL INJURIES

The incidence of tail tip injury was shown to increase on slatted floors compared with deep bedding packs[10,13] and on slatted floor compared with solid floor systems.[11,12] An investigation of health status of finishing beef cattle at 29 farms[15] found that bedding use was associated with a 33% reduction in culling risk compared with slatted pens. Sundrum and Rubelowski[16] surveyed 50 farms and found that farms that raised bulls on slatted floors reported greater mortality losses than those using deep-litter housing. From a cattle health and welfare perspective, these detrimental consequences provide support for the need to investigate intervention strategies to mitigate animal health and welfare concerns in these facilities.

Previous work by the author has looked at the consequences of tail docking in cattle housed in ICFs. Tail docking is a management practice that occurs in areas of the

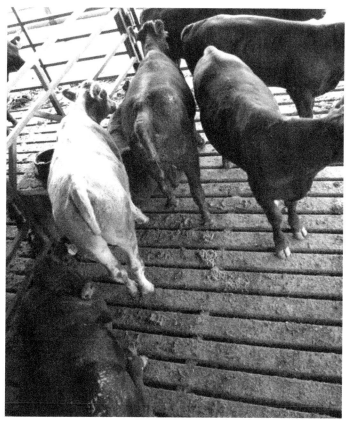

Fig. 2. Example of a slatted floor ICF.

midwest United States in confined, slatted floor feedlots. A survey of Michigan producers found that 50% of slatted floor farms routinely dock tails of cattle to reduce tail tip injuries and lameness and improve performance.[17] We recently completed studies with the primary objectives of determining the effect of tail docking on performance, carcass traits, and health parameters of feedlot cattle after tail docking of animals raised in slatted floor ICFs.[18] Three separate trials were performed. Trial 1 consisted of 140 Angus-cross (370-kg) yearling steers that spent 150 days on feed (DOF). Trial 2 consisted of 137 Angus-cross (255-kg) weaned steers that spent 232 DOF. Trial 3 consisted of 103 Holstein steers that weighed 370 kg at start of trial and spent 200 DOF. Cattle were randomly assigned to 1 of 2 treatment groups: tail docked or control. Performance parameters collected included daily gain, final weight, feed intake, and feed efficiency. Carcass quality data were collected at slaughter. Morbidity, mortality, incidence of lameness, and incidence of tail lesions were recorded. Across all 3 trials, there was no significant effect of treatment on performance parameters, carcass traits, or lameness (**Tables 1** and **2**). In all 3 trials, tail tip injuries occurred in 60% to 76% of undocked calves, as a result of living in the slatted floor environment, compared with tail tip injuries in 100% of docked calves, resulting from the tail docking procedure.

We were unable to identify a performance or significant health advantage to tail docking. However, tail tip injuries still occur in cattle raised in slatted floor ICFs.

Table 1
Health parameters of control and tail-docked cattle on slatted floors in 3 trials

| Item[a] | Trial[b] | Treatment Groups | | P value |
		Control[c]	Docked[c]	
Morbidity	1	8 (70)	3 (69)	.12
	2	20 (69)	21 (68)	.81
	3	15 (56)	9 (56)	.17
Lameness	1	8 (70)	2 (69)	.05
	2	3 (69)	4 (68)	.68
	3	9 (56)	6 (56)	.37

[a] Morbidity and lameness were diagnosed according to farm protocol by farm personnel.
[b] Trials: trial 1, backgrounded Angus-cross steers; trial 2, weaned Angus-cross calves; trial 3, backgrounded Holstein steers.
[c] Number of cases (number of animals per group).
Adapted from Kroll LK, Grooms DL, Siegford J, et al. Effects of tail docking on health and performance of beef cattle in confined, slatted floor feedlots. J Animal Sci 2014;92:4108–14; with permission.

Because of the animal welfare issues associated with tail docking and tail injuries, we recommend pursuing alternative solutions to reducing the incidence of tail tip injury in feedlot cattle housed in slatted floor ICFs.

We have also looked at behavior of feedlot cattle that have been tail docked and reported that cattle show behavior consistent with acute pain after tail docking and long-term fly irritation.[19] This finding is consistent with similar work performed in dairy cattle (reviewed by Kroll and colleagues[19]). As an example, in calves with docked tails, there

Table 2
Performance parameters of tail-docked and control cattle on slatted floors in 3 trials

| Item | Trial[a] | Treatment Groups | | P value |
		Control	Docked	
Number of cattle	1	70	70	—
	2	69	68	—
	3	51	52	—
Initial body weight (kg)	1	369.8	369.1	.96
	2	244.5	264.8	.14
	3	404.8	403.5	.97
Final body weight (kg)	1	611.7	611.4	.93
	2	584.6	599.7	.29
	3	651.9	665.9	.50
Overall average daily gain (kg/d)	1	1.51	1.51	.94
	2	1.47	1.44	.62
	3	1.33	1.40	.27
Overall gain to feed ratio	1	0.146	0.147	.94
	2	0.173	0.167	.22
	3	0.113	0.116	.57

[a] Trials: trial 1, backgrounded Angus-based steers, DOF 150; trial 2, weaned Angus-based calves, DOF 232; trial 3, backgrounded Holstein steers, DOF 200.
Adapted from Kroll LK, Grooms DL, Siegford J, et al. Effects of tail docking on health and performance of beef cattle in confined, slatted floor feedlots. J Animal Sci 2014;92:4108–14; with permission.

is a significant increase in step counts after tail docking, which lasts for at least 12 days.[19] There are several possible reasons for this increased activity. First, removal of the tail partly takes away ability to avoid flies, causing the calves to walk or stomp to physically move away from or dislodge flies. Our study was intentionally conducted in the summer months, when fly numbers were high, to specifically observe behaviors associated with fly irritation. Walking activity has been shown to be significantly increased in yearling feedlot steers under high levels of fly burden.[20] Second, increased activity in the tail-docked cattle may be caused by either acute or chronic pain associated with the tail amputation procedure.

Although these initial studies have answered some questions regarding the specific practice of tail docking, they also showed knowledge gaps related to animal welfare aspects of ICFs, which has spurred the need for ongoing evaluation of modern feedlot housing systems and the management strategies used in them.

LAMENESS IN CATTLE HOUSED IN INDOOR CONFINED FEEDLOTS

Lameness is the second most important health issue in fed cattle, regardless of housing system.[21] The problem is also a persistent one, because the reported incidence of lameness in feedlots has changed little in the past 10 years (**Fig. 3**). Lameness is particularly problematic for feedlot cattle housed in ICFs, because they often incorporate concrete slatted flooring.[7–9] Forty-two percent of the feedlots in Michigan, a key cattle-feeding state in the eastern corn belt, are slatted floor facilities, a type of ICF.[17]

In contrast to dairy cattle, there is little information in the literature about feedlot lameness. When a PubMed search is performed using the term feedlot lameness, a total of 8 references are cited (conducted by D.L.G., March 6, 2014). There is more information available on specific disease conditions, but little as it relates to feedlots in general, and even less as it relates to ICFs. Reports on the causes of lameness in feedlot cattle suggest that problems involving the foot are most common and include

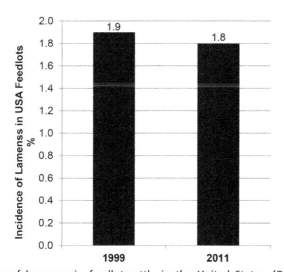

Fig. 3. Incidence of lameness in feedlot cattle in the United States. (*Data from* USDA. Feedlot 2011 "Part IV: Health and health management on U.S. feedlots with a capacity of 1000 or more head" USDA–APHIS–VS–CEAH–NAHMS. Literature Review on the Welfare Implications of Tail Docking of Cattle. Fort Collins (CO): AVMA; 2014.)

foot rot, toe abscesses and mechanical injuries.[22,23] However, these reports are focused more on feedlot cattle housed in outdoor dry lots typical of the Great Plains and western US feedlot industry and may not represent what is commonly seen in ICFs. As an example, field reports and personal observations of lameness issues in upper midwest ICFs indicate that lameness problems such as papillomatous digital dermatitis (heel warts) and polyarthritis may be more common than foot rot and toe abscesses (D.L.G., personal observation and personal correspondence with Drs Arnold Hentschl and Jan Shearer, 2014). As mentioned earlier, researchers have correlated slatted floors, a common flooring type in ICFs, to an increased risk of lameness in feedlot cattle.[8,9] However, characterization of other risk factors, such as breed, age, DOF, stocking density, and so forth, has not been studied in slatted floor ICFs.

Strategies to mitigate lameness in ICFs have not been scientifically evaluated. The use of rubber-covered slatted floors has been introduced to the US feedlot industry; however, no significant data have been gathered in typical US feeding situations to measure potential benefit of this intervention.

In dairy cattle, lameness has been more extensively studied. As expected, the environment has a major influence on lameness.[24,25] Multiple studies[26–28] have shown that cattle housed on solid concrete or slatted concrete floors have higher incidence of lameness and claw disorders. When slatted floors are rubberized, the incidence of lameness is decreased.[28,29]

Lameness in swine housed on concrete slats has also been examined. Similar to dairy cattle, flooring is one of the main features of the swine environment that affects lameness.[30,31] Some research exists on the use of rubber slat mats in sow housing. Tuyttens and colleagues[32] and Elmore and colleagues[33] reported welfare benefits for group-housed sows on rubber slat mats, such as lower body lesion scores and greater ease of changing posture. In a more recent study, Calderón Díaz and colleagues[34] reported that rubber-coated slats decreased lameness in sows, although they did increase the risk of claw lesions.

RISK OF PATHOGEN SPREAD

Because of the nature of how feedlots are managed and cattle are acquired, pathogens are ubiquitous in feedlots in the United States. Because of the close confinement of the cattle, pathogen transmission is more likely in an ICF, and therefore, disease dynamics may be different from those seen in open lot outdoor feedlots common in the western United States. With respect to respiratory disease, the most important disease of feedlot cattle, airborne pathogen concentration is a function of many factors, including type of animal (age, breed, sex), housing system, stocking density, bedding, humidity, dust particle density and size, noxious gas concentrations (eg, methane, carbon dioxide) and frequency of air exchanges (ventilation). Improved ventilation is 1 important means whereby airborne pathogen concentration can be decreased; however, pathogen removal is not a linear function, and practical as well as theoretic limits are often observed.[35] As the airborne pathogen load increases, ventilation provides progressively less protection against respiratory pathogen transmission. Stocking rate has a greater effect on airborne pathogen density than ventilation.[35,36] As an example, a 2-fold increase in stocking density requires nearly a 10-fold increase in ventilation to maintain the same airborne pathogen density.[36] So, because of the high stocking density of ICFs, pathogen loads are naturally increased, and can be exacerbated with poorly ventilated systems. Similarly, other pathogens commonly found in feedlots, such as Coccidia, may be transmitted faster in high-density ICFs.

OTHER HEALTH HAZARDS

Rapid deaths from exposure to high concentrations of hydrogen sulfide (H_2S) gas related to agitation of manure stored under ICFs has been reported in cattle.[37] H_2S is a highly toxic gas produced by the anaerobic decomposition of sulfur-containing organic matter. It is frequently associated with the breakdown of manure in storage pits. Because of the low solubility of H_2S in water, much of the gas is trapped in bubbles in the manure. Agitation of the manure pit before removal by pumping can release the gas, resulting in a rapid increase in H_2S to lethal concentrations in the confinement facility.

ANIMAL WELFARE CONSIDERATIONS

Concerns about animal welfare in intensively housed livestock systems have certainly been expressed and have led to changes in housing systems in both the poultry and swine industry. ICFs have not received the scrutiny that other livestock systems have received. However, this does not mean that there are no potential welfare concerns. Certainly, animals housed in close confinement in other livestock industries are viewed as having poor animal welfare, so there is no reason to believe this may not happen in the beef feedlot industry as well. Tail docking to control injuries in ICFs raises concern from the aspect of animal welfare because of the possibility of pain, both acute[38,39] and chronic,[40] increased fly burden from a shortened tail,[41,42] and loss of a method for communication between cattle.[43] The topic of tail docking has been addressed by many professional associations and industry groups. Based on current literature, the American Veterinary Medical Association (AVMA) and American Association of Bovine Practitioners both have position statements that oppose the routine tail docking of cattle.[44,45] The AVMA further specifies that tails should be docked only in cases in which tail removal is a curative procedure, and the procedure must be performed by a licensed veterinarian.[46] Other potential welfare issues that should be examined include discomfort and lameness, which may accompany standing and lying on concrete floors, and high stocking densities, which could limit movement and normal lying positions.

SUMMARY

ICFs offer advantages that make them desirable in northern climates where high rainfall and snowfall occur. These facilities increase the risk of certain health risks, including lameness and tail injuries. Closed confinement can also facilitate the rapid spread of infectious disease. Veterinarians can help to manage these health risks by implementing management practices to reduce their occurrence.

REFERENCES

1. FASS. Guide for the care and use of agricultural animals in agricultural research and teaching. Consortium for developing a guide for the care and use of agricultural animals in agricultural research and teaching. 3rd edition. Champaign (IL): Federation of Animal Science Societies; 2010.
2. Rust SR. Facilities for feeding Holstein and beef cattle. In: Managing and marketing quality Holstein steers proceedings. Ames (IA): Iowa State University Extension and Outreach; 2005. Available at: http://www.extension.iastate.edu/dairy team/managing-marketing-quality-holstein-steers-proceedings. Accessed January 10, 2015.

3. Standorf D, Metz K, Rust SR. Comparison of facility type and time on feed on growth and carcass characteristics of growing-finishing steers, vol. 575. East Lansing (MI): Mich. State Univ. Beef Cattle, Sheep Forage Res. Dem. Rep; 2001. p. 54–9.

4. Farlin SD. Beef confinement vs. open lot feeding. Lincoln (NE): Nebraska Beef Cattle Rep; 1974. EC 74–218:13.

5. Vetter RL, Geasler MR, Mobley E, et al. Feedlot performance and production costs of cattle fed on slotted-floor-cold-confinement vs. outside mounded lots. Ames (IA): Iowa State Univ. Beef Cattle Res.A.S; 1971. p. R150.

6. Harrison JD and Smith DR. Manure storage selection, Utah state extension. 2004. Available at: http://extension.usu.edu/files/factsheets/AG-AWM-01-3.pdf. Accessed January 10, 2015.

7. Hickey MC, Earley B, Fisher AD. The effect of floor type and space allowance on welfare indicators of finishing steers. Ir J Agric Food Res 2003;44:89–100.

8. Westerath HS, Gygax L, Mayer C, et al. Leg lesions and cleanliness of finishing bulls kept in housing systems with different lying area surfaces. Vet J 2007; 174:77–85.

9. Graunke KL, Telezhenko E, Hessle A, et al. Does rubber flooring improve welfare and production in growing bulls in fully slatted floor pens? Anim Welf 2011;20: 173–83.

10. Madsen EB, Nielsen K. A study of tail tip necrosis in young fattening bulls on slatted floors. Nord Vet Med 1885;37:349–57.

11. Drolia H, Luescher UA, Meek AH. Tail-tip necrosis in Ontario feedlot cattle–2 case-control studies. Prev Vet Med 1990;9:195–205.

12. Drolia H, Luescher UA, Meek AH, et al. Tail tip necrosis in Ontario beef feedlot cattle. Can Vet J 1991;32:23–9.

13. Schrader L, Roth HR, Winterling C, et al. The occurrence of tail tip alterations in fattening bulls kept under different husbandry conditions. Animal Welf 2001;10: 119–30.

14. Thomson DU, Taylor W, Noffsinger T, et al. Tail tip necrosis in a confined cattle feeding operation. Bovine Practitioner 2009;43:18–22.

15. Cerchiaro I, Contiero B, Mantovani R. Analysis of factors affecting health status of animals under intensive beef production systems. Ital J Anim Sci 2005;4: 122–4.

16. Sundrum A, Rubelowski I. The meaningfulness of design criteria in relation to the mortality of fattening bulls. Acta Agric Scand A Anim Sci 2001;51:48–52.

17. Miller SR. Survey of tail docking procedures of Michigan livestock producers. East Lansing (MI): Michigan Agricultural Experiment Station, Center for Economic Analysis; 2010. p. 1–14.

18. Kroll LK, Grooms DL, Siegford J, et al. Effects of tail docking on health and performance of beef cattle in confined, slatted floor feedlots. J Animal Sci 2014;92: 4108–14.

19. Kroll LK, Grooms DL, Siegford J, et al. Effects of tail docking on behavior of confined feedlot cattle. J Animal Sci 2014;92(10):4701–10.

20. Harvey TL, Launchbaugh JL. Effect of horn flies on behavior of cattle. J Econ Entomol 1982;75:25–7.

21. USDA. APHIS:VS. feedlot 2011 part IV: health and health management on US feedlots with a capacity of 1,000 or more head. Fort Collins (CO): USDA: APHIS:VS, CEAH, National Animal Health Monitoring System; 2013. Available at: http://www.aphis.usda.gov/animal_health/nahms/feedlot/downloads/feedlot2011/ Feed11_dr_PartIV.pdf. Accessed December 1, 2014.

22. Griffin D, Perino L, Hudson D. Feedlot lameness. G93-1159-A. Lincoln (NE): University of Nebraska Extension Bulletin; 1993. Available at: http://www.aabp.org/bmp_task_force/lameness/FeedlotLamenessGriffin.pdf. Accessed December 5, 2014.

23. Stokka GL, Lechtenberg K, Edwards T, et al. Lameness in feedlot cattle. Vet Clin North Am Food Anim Pract 2001;17:189–207.

24. Bergsten C. Effects of conformation and management system on hoof and leg diseases and lameness in dairy cows. Vet Clin North Am Food Anim Pract 2001;17:1–23.

25. Cook NB, Nordlund KV. The influence of the environment on dairy cow behavior, claw health and herd lameness dynamics. Vet J 2009;179:360–9.

26. Sogstad ÅM, Fjeldaas T, Østerås O, et al. Prevalence of claw lesions in Norwegian dairy cattle housed in tie stalls and free stalls. Prev Vet Med 2005;70: 191–209.

27. Rouha-Mülleder C, Iben C, Wagner E, et al. Relative importance of factors influencing the prevalence of lameness in Austrian cubicle loose-housed dairy cows. Prev Vet Med 2009;92:123–33.

28. Fjeldaas T, Sogstad AM, Osterås O. Locomotion and claw disorders in Norwegian dairy cows housed in freestalls with slatted concrete, solid concrete, or solid rubber flooring in the alleys. J Dairy Sci 2011;94:1243–55.

29. Platz S, Ahrens F, Bendel J, et al. What happens with cow behavior when replacing concrete slatted floor by rubber coating: a case study. J Dairy Sci 2008;91: 999–1004.

30. Spoolder HM, Geudeke MJ, Van der Peet-Schwering CM, et al. Group housing of sows in early parity: a review of success and risk factors. Livest Sci 2009;125:1–14.

31. Zurbrigg K, Blackwell T. Injuries, lameness, and cleanliness of sows in four group-housing gestation facilities in Ontario. J Swine Health Prod 2006;14:202–6.

32. Tuyttens FM, Wouters F, Struelens E, et al. Synthetic lying mats may improve lying comfort of gestating sows. Appl Anim Behav Sci 2008;114:76–85.

33. Elmore MP, Garner JP, Johnson AK, et al. A flooring comparison: the impact of rubber mats on the health, behaviour, and welfare of group-housed sows at breeding. Appl Anim Behav Sci 2010;123:7–15.

34. Calderón Díaz JA, Fahey AG, Kilbride AL, et al. Longitudinal study of the effect of rubber slat mats on locomotory ability, body, limb and claw lesions, and dirtiness of group housed sows. J Anim Sci 2013;91:3940–54.

35. Nardell EA, Keegan J, Cheney SA, et al. Airborne infection: theoretical limits of protection achievable by building ventilation. Am Rev Respir Dis 1991;144:302–6.

36. Wathes CM, Jones CD, Webster AJ. Ventilation, air hygiene and animal health. Vet Rec 1983;113:554–9.

37. Hooser SB, Van Alstine W, Kiupel M, et al. Acute pit gas (hydrogen sulfide) poisoning in confinement cattle. J Vet Diagn Invest 2000;12:272–5.

38. Schreiner DA, Ruegg PL. Responses to tail docking in calves and heifers. J Dairy Sci 2002;85:3287–96.

39. Tom EM, Duncan IH, Widowski TM, et al. Effects of tail docking using a rubber ring with or without anesthetic on behavior and production of lactating cows. J Dairy Sci 2002;85:2257–65.

40. Eicher SD, Cheng HW, Sorrells AD, et al. Behavioral and physiological indicators of sensitivity or chronic pain following tail docking. J Dairy Sci 2006;89:3047–51.

41. Eicher SD, Morrow-Tesch JL, Albright JL, et al. Tail-docking alters fly numbers, fly-avoidance behaviors, and cleanliness, but not physiological measures. J Dairy Sci 2001;84:1822–8.

42. Eicher SD, Dailey JW. Indicators of acute pain and fly avoidance behaviors in Holstein calves following tail-docking. J Dairy Sci 2002;85:2850–8.

43. Kiley-Worthington M. The tail movements of ungulates, canids and felids with particular reference to their causation and function as displays. Behavior 1976; 56:69–115.

44. AABP. AABP position statement: tail docking. 2010. Available at: http://www. aabp.org/members/publications/pdfs/AABP%20Tail%20Docking.pdf. Accessed November 10, 2014.

45. AVMA. Literature review on the welfare implications of tail docking of cattle. 2014. Available at: https://www.avma.org/KB/Policies/Pages/Tail-Docking-of-Cattle.aspx. 2013. Accessed November10, 2014.

46. AVMA. Welfare implications of tail docking of cattle. 2013. Available at: https://www. avma.org/KB/Resources/Backgrounders/Documents/tail_docking_cattle_bg nd. pdf. Accessed November 10, 2014.

Feedlot Pharmaceutical Documentation
Protocols, Prescriptions, and Veterinary Feed Directives

Michael D. Apley, DVM, PhD

KEYWORDS

- Feedlot • Protocols • Prescriptions • Veterinary feed directive

KEY POINTS

- Treatment protocols only work when based on sound case definitions, which serve as training guides for personnel who will apply the treatment regimens.
- Case definitions are necessary for both treatment eligibility and determination of success or failure at the end of the treatment protocol or the posttreatment interval (PTI).
- Treatment regimens contained in the protocol must be consistently applied if records are to be used for evaluation of outcomes.
- Protocols should also address methods for assuring that no animals enter the food chain with a violative drug residue.
- Prescriptions and veterinary feed directives (VFDs) are the official records of veterinary authorization of drug use by clients.

INTRODUCTION

In the new era of transparency in agricultural production, the days of oral treatment protocols and loosely associated authorizations for the use of drugs in food animals are gone. No longer do animals disappear into the next stage of the production system without being traced. Veterinarians are increasing the detail and complexity of treatment protocols in an effort to more precisely guide therapeutic interventions as well as documenting what was authorized. The triad of treatment protocols, prescriptions, and VFDs will soon guide all uses of medically important antimicrobials in food animals except for a few over-the-counter (OTC) products not administered in feed or water. Veterinarians will not only be responsible for these antimicrobial uses in food animals but also be accountable. In this environment, it is wise to develop a systematic

The author has nothing to disclose.
Department of Clinical Sciences, College of Veterinary Medicine, Kansas State University, 1800 Denison Avenue, Manhattan, KS 66506, USA
E-mail address: mapley@vet.ksu.edu

approach to documenting authorized treatments, defining how animals are selected for these treatments, and having a systematic method for documenting authorizations for drug use in client animals.

TREATMENT PROTOCOLS

Protocol sophistication will vary depending on the autonomy of the individuals treating cattle. Regardless of how extensive a protocol is, it is important that all the people who will be using it have ownership in developing the contents, monitoring results, and updating the protocol. The protocol becomes the pivotal document in crew training and documentation/discussion of treatment processes. Discussions of changes to the protocol should be readily entered into, but deviation from the protocol without mutually agreed alterations and a resulting change in the protocol should not be tolerated.

In addition to benefits to the production facility, detailed protocols and records of education and agreement related to the protocols are very important to the veterinarian in the case of a violative drug residue or regulatory inspection. Documenting a treatment strategy in a written protocol also serves as a "say it out loud to yourself" test for practicality and evidence-based status.

A complete feedlot protocol should include the diseases listed in **Box 1**. For some of these diseases (eg, respiratory disease, footrot), regimens are required for the early/middle feeding period as well as close to slaughter, where altered regimens prioritizing drugs with short withdrawal times become a priority. The written treatment protocol requires several basic inclusions to allow consistent application of treatments and evaluation of what happens after these treatments are administered:

- Characterization of the disease to be treated (case definitions)
- Treatment regimens
- Outcome definitions (success/failure)
- Animal disposition based on therapeutic outcome
- Methods for assuring that animals are not shipped with violative residues
- Signatures of the veterinarian authorizing the purchases and the owner/agent committing to using these drugs as authorized by the veterinarian

An example of a treatment protocol for low-risk respiratory disease is presented in **Box 2**.

Case Definitions

This term can induce eye rolls because it sounds rather academic, but creating a consistent case definition is the ideal strategy for agreeing, and then training, on selecting diseased animals for treatment. In feedlot protocols, there are 2 questions to be answered when creating a case definition. First, what characteristics of an animal cause it to be removed from the pen (pulled) for further evaluation? Second, what confirmatory tests are to be applied in the treatment facility to make the final decision to treat or not to treat?

Using respiratory disease as an example, depression is a primary component of the first stage. Other signs such as sunken flanks (an indicator of appetite), nasal and ocular discharge, and respiratory character may also be included. Sometimes it is hard for experienced and competent pen riders to put into words exactly what it is that makes them pull an animal for respiratory disease. Putting together a scoring system is an exercise that forces the reduction of visual cues into words, and the resulting discussions related to the appropriate scores for animals in the pen serve to hone the observational skills of newcomers (and maybe the experienced ones too).

Box 1
List of diseases that should be included in complete feedlot treatment protocol

Respiratory disease

    Low risk (expected morbidity <10%, case fatality 1%–2%)

    High risk (expected morbidity ≥10%, case fatality >2% up to 10%)

    Heavy cattle in close proximity to scheduled slaughter (usually 30–45 days), withdrawal times are now a primary consideration

    Acute interstitial pneumonia

    Tracheal edema (honkers)

    Diphtheria

Gastrointestinal disease

    Acidosis

    Bloat

    Coccidiosis

Musculoskeletal disease

    Footrot

    Toe and sole abscesses

    Undifferentiated lameness (eg, sprains)

    Hairy heel wart (strawberry footrot)

Central nervous system disease

    Polioencephalomalacia

    Thrombolic meningoencephalitis

    Listeriosis

    Nervous coccidiosis

Miscellaneous

    Rectal, vaginal, and uterine prolapses

    Calvers and abortions

    Anaphylactic shock

    Bullers

    Pink eye

    Abscesses

A common system includes a range of 0 to 4, with 0 being healthy and 4 denoting an animal unable to rise. **Table 1** outlines 1 set of verbal cues for the scores, but the best procedure would be for a veterinarian and the crew to develop their own. Progress has been made if the in-pen debates are typically centered on differences of 1 score. Other descriptions of the scores are (1) an early pull, arguments are valid on whether it is actually sick or not, (2) everyone ought to agree on this one, and (3) the calf is very ill and could have been pulled yesterday.

The second case definition stage for respiratory disease involves examination in the chute, which typically involves rectal temperature and/or lung auscultation. The author has witnessed systems ranging from treating every animal pulled to the approach of

---

Box 2
Example treatment guidelines

Respiratory Disease Example Protocol: For low-risk cattle where less than 10% morbidity and a case fatality rate of 1% to 2% are expected

Case definition for initial treatment:

In the pen: The primary sign is depression (moves slowly, hanging head, drooping ears, knuckling of hind fetlocks) and the animal may also display nasal discharge, sunken flanks, and increased respiratory effort. Diarrhea and ocular discharge may also be present.

At the chute: A minimum rectal temperature of 104°F (40°C) is required for therapy. Cattle without the minimum required rectal temperature should be evaluated for causes of not eating such as pen environment or acidosis.

Treatments:

Low-risk treatment #1: slaughter withdrawal 20 days

Day 0 Antibiotic 1: 3 mL/100 lb (1 ml/15 kg) subcutaneously in the neck, 16-gauge, 0.75-in needle, maximum of 10 mL/site with a handsbreadth distance between sites, return to home pen as soon as possible

Days 1–6: Observe only, cattle reaching a depression score of 4 should be humanely euthanized

Day 7: Observe and apply success or failure criteria

Case definition for success/failure determination: Cattle classified as treatment successes are displaying no signs of depression. Determining rectal temperature is not necessary if the animal seems clinically normal. Cattle displaying signs of depression should be brought to the treatment facility for determination of rectal temperature. Those with a rectal temperature of 104°F, or with a depression score of 2 or 3 regardless of the rectal temperature are to be moved to treatment #2. Those with a depression score of 1 and a rectal temperature of 104.0 F or less are to be returned to the home pen without treatment.

Low-risk treatment #2: slaughter withdrawal 30 days

Day 0 Antibiotic 1: 2 mL/100 lb (1 ml/23 kg) subcutaneously in the neck, 16-gauge, 0.75-in needle, maximum of 10 mL/site with a handsbreadth distance between sites, opposite side of the neck from treatment #1, return to home pen as soon as possible

Days 1–6: Observe only, cattle reaching a depression score of 4 should be humanely euthanized

Day 7: Observe and apply success/failure criteria, repeat treatment #2 for treatment failures and place in convalescent pen. Successes are returned to the home pen. Treatment failures are evaluated in the convalescent pen at 30 days and either returned to the home pen or sold as a realizer.

---

precise cutoffs based on rectal temperature. The philosophies for these approaches range from leaning toward minimizing the chance of missing even 1 calf that could benefit from treatment (the former) to a systematic approach to avoiding unwarranted treatment and therefore unnecessary cost and antimicrobial exposure (the latter). The strategy for determining this second stage cutoff also depends on how the first stage definitions are applied in the pen. Not the least of considerations for the second stage cutoffs is how many "buddies" accompany legitimate pulls to the treatment facilities based on the skill and commitment of the pen riders in bringing cattle out of the pen.

There can be some politics in the relationship between pen riders and the treatment crew if a feedlot is large enough for separate crews. Agreeing on a protocol for how each crew evaluates the cattle can ease some of the strain.

Table 1
Example description of clinical illness scores for respiratory cases in feedlots

Depression Score	Clinical Signs
0	Normal, no signs of depression
1	Slower than pen mates but still perks up when approached and does not appear weak; actively follows your movements with a raised head
2	Stands with head lowered, will perk up when approached but will return to depressed stance, moves slowly and falls toward back of group, may display signs of weakness such as incoordination
3	Obviously very weak, difficulty in moving with group, raises head only when approached closely
4	Moribund, unable to rise

Treatment Regimens

The intricacies of evidence for specific therapeutic decisions in feedlot treatment regimens are beyond the scope of this article. However, the veterinarian is expected to have a reason for inclusions in the treatment protocols. An argument against evidence-based protocols is often that the evidence simply does not exist either to support or to discourage inclusion of different treatment options; this approach may be used to justify inclusion of various drugs in protocols based on clinical impression or experience.

In the author's opinion, sometimes decrying the lack of data is because of the lack of looking. Evidence is available for many aspects of feedlot therapeutics. The effects of antibiotics on the outcome of bovine respiratory disease (BRD) therapy in feedlot animals as well as the analysis of comparative trials between the multiple antimicrobial options for this purpose have been well described.[1,2] Evidence for the effects of treatment for control of BRD has also been summarized.[3] The available data for ancillary therapy for BRD have been reviewed, and in spite of the positive publication bias of the literature, the evidence was found to be equivocal to discouraging.[4]

The evidence for individual animal therapy for footrot and hairy heel wart has also been reviewed, with clear evidence for the efficacy of some treatments.[5] Therapy for polioencephalomalacia has been evaluated, finding no clinical trial data for cattle; however, evaluation of other data found support for the use of thiamine and possibly for legal forms of dimethyl sulfoxide, while suggesting great caution in using dexamethasone or nonsteroidal antiinflammatory drugs because of the significant potential to cause harm.[6]

Despite differences in opinion on reasonable treatment protocol inclusions, there should be general agreement on what is necessary to properly document the protocol. A goal is that someone new to the facility is able to rapidly pick up the specifics of the protocol and apply them.

- Dose: Converted to mL/100 lb, mL/kg, or appropriate units. The specific concentration of the product should be specified if more than one is available. Production systems with computerized treatment systems and electronic scales are at an advantage in facilitating more precise dose determination for each animal.
- Route: This not only includes description of the route (eg, subcutaneous, intramuscular, topical, intravenous) but also the correct needle size and length and volume per site. The veterinarian may wish to also specify the appropriate injection equipment for each drug.

- Frequency: This may be as simple as once or may include periodic administrations.
- Duration: This category requires that the veterinarian determine when it is appropriate to evaluate treatment outcome and whether the animal should receive additional therapy or treatment should be discontinued. For a multiple injection drug, evaluation is often 24 hours after the last injection; however, the veterinarian may give more time for recovery before designating that a success or failure determination be made, similar to the PTI after single-injection drugs.
- Withdrawal time: Herein lies the reward for adhering to label regimens, the surety of a label withdrawal time. In other cases, the Food Animal Residue Avoidance Databank (FARAD) should be consulted.[7] In cases of extralabel drug use, the veterinarian is responsible for assuring that violative residues do not enter the food chain by assigning an appropriate exaggerated withdrawal time.

Time references in protocols have the potential to be misleading. For example, if a drug is given on Monday at 11:00 AM and it is to be evaluated on day 3, what does that mean? To some, 3 days may mean 3 periods of 24 hours each, whereby the day of administration is day 0 and the drug results would be evaluated on Thursday. To some, the day of administration is day 1, so the results should be evaluated on day 3, which is Wednesday. For this reason, shorter periods should be indicated by hours (eg, 24 hours) and longer periods expressed in days should be clarified in that the day of administration is either day 0 or day 1.

Volume per site is an important control point for injectable drugs. Some drugs have label indications, whereas rules for others are guided by quality assurance principles. Instructions should be clear as to splitting volumes in cases such as where the maximum volume per site is 15 mL and the dose is 17 mL. Also, the protocol should specify the distance between injection sites and what should happen when different drug regimens are concurrently administered and require multiple sites over a period of days. The author's rule is that it is time to carefully consider the treatment regimen when one starts to run out of injection sites. The protocol should be written in lay terms unless the veterinarian has educated the crew on definitions of specific terms.

Outcome Definitions

The animal has now been identified for treatment according to the case definition, the treatment regimen has been applied as per regimen, and it is time to decide the outcome. A veterinarian can dramatically affect the outcome distribution by how the success or failure definitions are constructed. For example, requiring the animal to meet the initial treatment criteria in order to be classified as a failure yields different treatment outcomes than requiring them to be normal in all categories before being classified as a success. The consequences of the criteria for initial treatment and success or failure ripple through the system by affecting relapse, mortality, and chronic disease rates.

Treatment outcome definitions must be readily measurable and have end points that can contribute to a definition. For example, a failure criteria of "have not satisfactorily responded" is a shortcut in protocol writing, which is not helpful. In contrast, defining depression score, lameness score, rectal temperature, or perhaps changes in body weight during the treatment period (if available) can give criteria that may then be altered in response to dissatisfaction with outcomes. The selection of definition criteria may also be heavily influenced by the skill sets of the personnel applying the definitions. In some systems, a definition heavily relying on depression scores may be appropriate, whereas others may need more objective measures. In the author's opinion, if an animal recovering from respiratory disease has a normal depression score and appears to be eating/drinking, the rectal temperature has as much potential to drive unnecessary additional therapy as it does to clarify success or failure.

The advent of single-injection drugs with the ability to immediately return animals to the home pen has kept go-home pens less populated but has also presented a challenge in applying success or failure definitions at the end of the PTI. Some feedlots have used chalk marks with the day of treatment or the day the animal is eligible for re-treatment (the end of the PTI). These dates may also be displayed on cards affixed to the forehead with tag cement, although retention and legibility may start to decrease toward the end of 10-day PTIs. Another option is to provide the pen riders with lists of treatment eligibility dates for individual tag numbers; this becomes an eligibility by exclusion system where animals' eligible dates are only evaluated if they appear to need further therapy. The goal is to provide a mechanism whereby animals in need of further treatment receive it as soon as possible after they are eligible; just having a hospital tag or a notched lot tag indicates that the animal has been treated but not when, and the pen rider may try to "look them well" by giving them more time to respond to treatment well after they have become eligible for the next regimen.

Animal Disposition

Disposition for treatment successes is relatively easy: send them to the home pen or leave them if they are already in the home pen. For failures, it can be more complicated. The protocol should specify hospital pen or convalescent pen destinations as well as the next step in treatment. It is also the responsibility of the veterinarian to specify when humane euthanasia is appropriate and to work with the crew to identify those animals requiring euthanasia.

Assuring Violative Residues Do Not Occur

Larger feedlots with computerized records typically have a component of these record systems, such as a shipping report, which checks to see if any cattle in that lot still have a withdrawal time in effect at the time of shipment to slaughter. In these cases, the veterinarian should be part of determining the plan to assure this is done before shipment for each lot. Some feedlots have a requirement that this report be printed, signed, and placed in the lot file before shipment. Examining this report when the cattle are already loaded or heading down the road does little good. Under no circumstances should an animal with a withdrawal time still in effect be allowed to enter the food chain. Cattle may be sold (not for slaughter) with a drug withdrawal still in effect, but a notice of the remaining withdrawal period must accompany the cattle and be delivered to the buyer.

Another responsibility of the veterinarian in avoiding violative drug residues is to construct separate protocols for cattle nearing slaughter (typically within 30 to 45 days). Drugs with short withdrawal times should be prioritized in these situations if possible.

In the case of extralabel use, the veterinarian is required by regulation to assign an extended slaughter withdrawal time that assures that no violative residues enter the food chain.[8] In the case of drugs with no tolerance in the edible tissues of the food animal, any detected drug is violative. If this information is not available, and the withdrawal time cannot be assigned, then the animal or animals must not enter the food chain. The standard for determining if evidence is available to establish an exaggerated slaughter withdrawal time is the FARAD.[7]

Protocol Signatures and Availability

Signatures of the veterinarian and the owner/authorized agent demonstrate that the protocol was provided and reviewed on a specific date. These signatures also document the agreement of the owner/agent to abide by the protocol inclusions. This agreement can be specified under the owner/agent signature blank. Both parties should date their signatures and retain a signed copy for reference. The visit report of the veterinarian should document each time training occurs in relation to the treatment protocol, as well as any authorized deviations from the protocol.

The final protocol should be available in treatment facilities. Computer guidelines that are accessed during treatment might not include specifics such as volume per site or needle size, so the full hard-copy version of the protocol needs to be within reach.

Applying Treatment Protocols

It is just not possible to accurately evaluate a practice or procedure that is not consistently applied. Once the protocol has been established, monitoring for protocol drift and potential improvements are the new priorities. Monitoring involves going through treatment records on a periodic basis, either systematically or through spot checks. One effective way to monitor protocol adherence is to routinely review treatment histories of high-morbidity groups and mortalities. If protocols are not being followed, routine sampling catches this. Sometimes the more inventive derivations involve animals that appear to be in danger of mortality.

A challenge in working with personnel who implement the protocols is that sometimes those who have worked at other facilities may feel that the protocols used at other locations are more effective. In these cases, the challenge is balancing the participation of that individual in the protocol development process with holding the line for adherence to the attending veterinarian's judgment. These situations underscore the importance of ownership of the protocol by all involved in the implementation. In the author's experience, if the crew decides that the protocol is not effective, then it will not be efficacious.

It is important to recognize that the case fatality and treatment success rates observed from even the most faithfully applied protocols do not necessarily primarily reflect the effects of the drug or drugs. These measures of case outcomes are because of a combination of disease challenge, animal physiologic status (including immunity), and drug effect. Changes in the rates of case outcomes can be due to a change in the status of any component; therefore clinical impressions of changes in drug efficacy should be highly scrutinized.

PRESCRIPTIONS

Veterinarians have developed multiple methods for providing prescriptions to be filled by other entities that are entitled by law or regulation to dispense drugs on the order of a veterinarian. In addition to current prescription drugs, as of December, 2016, prescriptions will be required for all antimicrobials used in the water for food animals as described in Food and Drug Administration Center for Veterinary Medicine (FDA/CVM) Guidance for Industry (GFI) documents 209 and 213.[9,10] There will only be a limited selection of OTC injectable antimicrobials left for food animals. Some of these may be purchased as OTC products without a prescription, whereas some common extralabel uses of these antimicrobials require a prescription (eg, procaine penicillin G).

Prescription Inclusions

In writing prescriptions, there are reasonable inclusions that inform the dispenser and the end user, as well as protect the veterinarian (**Box 3**). Although an expiration date is

---

Box 3
Inclusions for prescriptions for feedlots

Name and contact information of the veterinarian

Name and contact information of the owner or authorized agent

Identification of drug or drugs

   Trade or generic name (including if generics are authorized)

   Specific concentration or content if appropriate

Container size or sizes authorized

Maximum number of containers of each authorized size

Approved use conditions

   "According to the label"

   Specific conditions for use

   "According to the treatment protocol"

Signature of the veterinarian

Signature of the owner/agent to whom the prescription is provided

Expiration date of the prescription

---

not required, it is a good option to force renewal of the prescription periodically so that use can be reviewed. This renewal could be carried out in concert with reviewing the treatment protocol. An expiration date on a prescription also limits the liability of the veterinarian if the veterinary-client-patient relationship (VCPR) is severed and the client continues to purchase drugs based on the prescription. In this case, the veterinarian may choose to send letters to drug dispensing entities that the VCPR is no longer in effect and therefore the prescription is no longer valid.

It is within the purview of the veterinarian to require that copies of invoices for drug purchases be provided so that awareness of drug use can be maintained. Limiting the amounts of drug that may be purchased during the authorized prescription period also provides a warning to the veterinarian that something is going on when either the drug distributor or client requests expansion of the prescription limits. For this reason, the amounts of drug authorized on the prescription should be carefully considered in order to provide a small buffer for unanticipated needs, while also setting a limit on extensive use, which may indicate a need for intervention on the part of the veterinarian.

State pharmacy laws may have a significant effect on the requirements of prescription writing, and the veterinarian is responsible for knowing these details. In some states, a purchase order is used and the drugs are drop-shipped directly to the client based on this order. A prescription is not required for dispensing directly from the veterinary practice to the client. However, when multiple people in the practice may be responsible for dispensing drugs to the client, it is reasonable that a list of drugs authorized for a client be available.

VETERINARY FEED DIRECTIVES

As described in GFI documents 209 and 213, in December, 2016, all labels of medically important antimicrobials for use in or on the feed of food animals will require that the drug only be used as authorized by a VFD.[9,10] At the time of this writing

(January 2015), the definition of medically important does not include the ionophores (eg, monensin, lasalocid), bacitracin, bambermycins, or pleuromutilins (eg, tiamulin). A veterinarian does not have to provide VFDs for the use of these nonmedically important antimicrobials.

This proposed VFD rule was released in December of 2013 concurrently with the release of the final GFI 213.[11] A 90-day comment period was established; the FDA/CVM gathered input through stakeholder meetings and other activities and is in the process of formulating the final rule at the time of this writing. It is apparent the proposed rule will closely approximate the final rule, but there are multiple fine points that await clarification. The reader is directed to updates and training from food animal veterinary organizations such as the American Association of Bovine Practitioners and Academy of Veterinary Consultants for continued guidance on how the final rule evolves and will affect bovine practice.

This proposed regulation has 5 key changes in the existing VFD regulation.

1. User-friendly reorganization of the VFD rule
2. Increased flexibility for licensed veterinarians issuing VFDs
   a. The current regulation requires veterinary supervision for a VFD to be written. The proposed regulation changes this to supervision or oversight.
   b. The proposed regulation removes the explicit VCPR provision and replaces it with the requirement that veterinarians ordering the use of VFD drugs must be "in compliance with all applicable veterinary licensing and practicing requirements." This requirement defers the VCPR standard to the veterinary profession and the individual states to determine the requirements of a valid VCPR.
   c. Veterinarians will be required to specify duration of use, approximate number of animals to be fed the medicated feed, and level of VFD drug in the feed. However, they will not be required to specify the amount of medicated feed to be dispensed.
3. Continued access to Category I type A medicated feed articles by unlicensed feed mills
   a. At present, a VFD drug is automatically a Category II medicated feed, which means that the type A feed article for that drug would only be available to the limited number of licensed feed mills. The proposed regulation would not require a VFD drug to automatically become a Category II medicated feed.
4. Increased flexibility for animal producers purchasing VFD feeds
5. Lower record-keeping burden for all involved parties
   a. Duration of record keeping is proposed to be dropped from 2 years to 1 year.

At the time of this writing, discussions related to how veterinarians will provide all these new VFDs as well as the requirements for a valid relationship between producers and veterinarians are taking place at the state level. The FDA/CVM made it clear in GFI #120 that "The term 'appropriately licensed' veterinarian, as it pertains to 21 CFR 558.6, means that the veterinarian has a valid license to practice veterinary medicine in the State in which the animals being treated are located."[12]

SUMMARY

An up-to-date and accurate treatment protocol, which is agreed to by both the veterinarian and the people who will carry it out, is essential to assuring that drugs will be used by clients and their employees in the manner directed by the veterinarian. In addition, accompanying prescriptions and VFDs complete the triad of assuring judicious use of drugs in food animals and documenting the instructions given by the veterinarian.

REFERENCES

1. DeDonder KD, Apley MD. A review of the expected effects of antimicrobials in bovine respiratory disease treatment and control using outcomes from published randomized clinical trials with negative controls. Vet Clin North Am Food Anim Pract 2015;31(1):97–111.
2. O'Connor AM, Coetzee JF, da Silva N, et al. A mixed treatment comparison meta-analysis of antibiotic treatments for bovine respiratory disease. Prev Vet Med 2013;110:77–87.
3. Nickell JS, White BJ. Metaphylactic antimicrobial therapy for bovine respiratory disease in stocker and feedlot cattle. Vet Clin North Am Food Anim Pract 2010; 26:285–301.
4. Francoz D, Buczinski S, Apley M. Evidence related to the use of ancillary drugs in bovine respiratory disease (Anti-inflammatory and others): are they justified or not? Vet Clin North Am Food Anim Pract 2012;28:23–38.
5. Apley MD. Clinical evidence for individual animal therapy of papillomatous digital dermatitis (hairy heel wart) and infectious bovine pododermatitis (foot rot). Vet Clin North Am Food Anim Pract 2015;31(1):81–95.
6. Apley MD. Consideration of evidence for therapeutic interventions in bovine polioencephalomalacia. Vet Clin North Am Food Anim Pract 2015;31(1):151–61.
7. Food Animal Residue Avoidance Databank. Available at: http://www.farad.org/. Accessed January 21, 2015.
8. Food and Drug Administration Center for Veterinary Medicine Final Rule. Extralabel Drug Use in Animals. Fed Regist 1996;61(217):57731–46.
9. Food and Drug Administration Center for Veterinary Medicine Guidance for Industry #209. The judicious use of medically important antimicrobial drugs in food-producing animals. 2012. Available at: http://www.fda.gov/downloads/AnimalVeterinary/GuidanceComplianceEnforcement/GuidanceforIndustry/UCM216936.pdf. Accessed January 21, 2015.
10. Food and Drug Administration Center for Veterinary Medicine Guidance for Industry #213. New animal drugs and new animal drug combination products administered in or on medi8cated feed or drinking water of food-producing animals: Recommendations for drug sponsors for voluntarily aligning product use conditions with GFI #209. Available at: http://www.fda.gov/downloads/AnimalVeterinary/GuidanceComplianceEnforcement/GuidanceforIndustry/UCM299624.pdf. Accessed January 21, 2015.
11. FDA takes significant steps to address antimicrobial resistance. Available at: http://www.fda.gov/AnimalVeterinary/NewsEvents/CVMUpdates/ucm378166.htm. Accessed July 28, 2014.
12. Guidance for Industry - Veterinary Feed Directive Regulation Questions and Answers Final Guidance. 2009. Available at: http://www.fda.gov/downloads/AnimalVeterinary/GuidanceComplianceEnforcement/GuidanceforIndustry/UCM0526BBBPMIKE0.pdf. Accessed July 28, 2014.

Index

Note: Page numbers of article titles are in **boldface** type.

Vet Clin Food Anim 31 (2015) 317–322
http://dx.doi.org/10.1016/S0749-0720(15)00034-1   vetfood.theclinics.com
0749-0720/15/$ – see front matter © 2015 Elsevier Inc. All rights reserved.

Moving?

Make sure your subscription moves with you!

To notify us of your new address, find your **Clinics Account Number** (located on your mailing label above your name), and contact customer service at:

Email: journalscustomerservice-usa@elsevier.com

800-654-2452 (subscribers in the U.S. & Canada)
314-447-8871 (subscribers outside of the U.S. & Canada)

Fax number: 314-447-8029

Elsevier Health Sciences Division
Subscription Customer Service
3251 Riverport Lane
Maryland Heights, MO 63043

*To ensure uninterrupted delivery of your subscription, please notify us at least 4 weeks in advance of move.

Printed and bound by CPI Group (UK) Ltd, Croydon, CR0 4YY

03/10/2024

01040465-0012